Simple Principles®
to Get Fit

Alex A. Lluch
Author of Over 3 Million Books Sold!

WS Publishing Group
San Diego, California

SIMPLE PRINCIPLES®
TO GET FIT

By Alex A. Lluch

Published by WS Publishing Group
San Diego, California 92119
Copyright © 2009 by WS Publishing Group

Designed by WS Publishing Group:
David Defenbaugh

For Inquiries:
Log on to www.WSPublishingGroup.com
E-mail info@WSPublishingGroup.com

ISBN13: 978-1-934386-09-5

Printed in China

TABLE OF CONTENTS

INTRODUCTION

Just about everyone has an image of what the perfect body looks like. Movies, television, and magazines bombard us every day with images of women with sculpted abdomens and men with bulging biceps. We see these pictures repeatedly and begin to believe that we should resemble this ideal. In order to reach what society has deemed the "perfect body," we subject ourselves to starvation diets and get-fit-quick schemes that serve only to compound our negative self-image and distance us from our goals. We risk our health and happiness trying to match an image that, for most of us, is unattainable, and we spend billions of dollars in doing so.

What we consider an ideal body continues to become thinner while Americans on the whole are getting larger. Just take a quick look at the cover of a fashion or entertainment magazine. The stars we revere are often far more slender than is really healthy. Yet, as the ideal gets slimmer; studies are showing that, since the mid-1980s, the rate of obesity in America is rapidly on the rise. As a matter of fact, we are facing an obesity epidemic that reaches across all gender, age, and racial lines, and this epidemic has resulted in a significant increase in obesity-related illnesses such as diabetes, heart disease, and strokes.

Although obesity is at epidemic levels, much of it is preventable, as it is simply the result of an unhealthy and inactive lifestyle. With work, school, family, and social commitments competing for our time, we tend to lose sight of the need for proper exercise and fitness. Our fast-paced way of life leads us to do what is easy and convenient, rather than doing those things that we know are good for us. All too often, it is our bodies that pay the price for this neglect.

In order to reverse the American obesity problem, we must make healthy eating and regular exercise a priority in our lives. This requires hard work and dedication, but the good news is that we need not pursue impossible ideals in order to make a real change. By focusing on daily achievement and personal improvement, we can take control of our lives and transform our minds and bodies.

Contributing to the obesity epidemic, and just as dangerous even when not obese, is leading a sedentary lifestyle. Recently researchers have been able to correlate the level of physical activity with the risk of dying. Results are astonishing. Lack of physical activity was attributed to 20 percent of all deaths of people 35 and older. This is more than can be attributed to smoking.

As many of us know, yet ignore, physical activity and healthy eating are a critical component in the health of the human body. As a matter of fact, the more you use your body and the better the fuel is that you supply it, the healthier it gets. However, many of us today buy empty-nutrition meals at fast-food drive-ups and then spend hours at home watching TV. Sitting at jobs behind a desk for hours a day, many of us are getting no physical activity whatsoever.

Though most of us understand that physical activity will make us stronger and healthier, we just don't take the time to exercise. If we did, we'd send oxygen in our muscles, tissues, and organs, improving our flexibility. We'd move fluids, especially lymph fluids and blood, and nutrients; we'd improve cellular respiration and our nervous systems. Our moods would improve and we'd see a reverse in a number of chronic disease, including breast and prostate cancer, type-2 diabetes, heart disease, osteoporosis, and more.

Is there any way we can get all these wonderful benefits without diet and exercise? No: The answer is we must dedicate ourselves to hard work. That's where *Simple Principles® to Get Fit* will help. This book will teach the secrets of combining physical fitness and nutrition to make permanent, healthy lifestyle changes.

What is this book about?

This book will teach you the basic principles of diet, exercise, and fitness and show you how to incorporate them into your daily life. These principles will change your current views toward fitness, enhance your understanding of nutrition, and explain how you can conquer your own unhealthy attitudes toward fitness.

You will learn how to examine your present fitness level and identify your personal goals. This book will show you how to create a personalized workout routine that is easy to follow, maintain, and enjoy. As a result you will improve your ability to train your body and unleash its hidden potential.

This book will inform you about the principles that can make you a healthier and happier individual. It does not contain any "get-fit-quick" remedies, but offers scientifically based information that will help you make lasting changes to your lifestyle.

This book will reveal principles to healthy eating and how diet affects your physical fitness and exercise routines. Study the following pages to learn to alter the way you think about health and fitness. You will learn to judge your progress based on your individual improvements and achievements, and you will begin to shift away from unrealistic societal expectations, to a more personal view of fitness.

It's time to throw out the old, "no pain, no gain" and "do-or-die" mentalities toward fitness. This book shows you how to judge your fitness levels based on effort and personal achievement and how to optimize your body's performance in an enjoyable manner through nutrition and exercise. You will learn how long-term physical exercise and healthy eating are both more beneficial and more sustainable than drastic get-fit-quick schemes. Fitness will cease to be overwhelming, but rather a pleasurable aspect of your life.

Who should read this book?

Simple Principles® to Get Fit is designed for anyone looking to improve his or her physical fitness. The principles included in this book apply to all of us, no matter what our current or goal fitness levels are. No matter what your age is, this book will show you how you can improve your quality of life by eating right, keeping well-hydrated, and exercising regularly.

This book is ideal for those just starting a fitness routine as well as for those looking to create a more sustainable path to fitness. It will prepare you to make lasting changes in your personal fitness by focusing on the key principles of success.

This book is intended for those who are interested in designing a well-balanced exercise plan for themselves. It will show you the 3 components of fitness, cardiovascular, strength, and flexibility training, while giving you the hows and whys for each. By defining the different components of training, and discussing the importance of each one to your program, you'll learn how to train for optimal performance and better overall physical fitness.

This book is made for those who want to understand the defining role that our food choices have on the health and fitness of our bodies. It will describe the mounting evidence that says that our bodies have specific nutritional requirements that promote our fitness advances, make us less prone to disease, and bolster our metabolisms.

In conclusion, many of us spend less time maintaining our bodies than we do our cars or homes. This book will show you how to adopt and maintain a healthy lifestyle that pays attention to nutrition and physical exercise. You will see that even minor changes to your lifestyle can help you significantly improve your level of fitness and overall quality of life.

Why should you read this book?

Simple Principles® to Get Fit will help you make positive changes in your life. You will gain self-confidence when you improve your physical fitness through diet and exercise. Your success will spill over into other aspects of your life, resulting in an overall increase in your happiness and contentment.

You should read this book to set a healthy example for your children. Studies have shown that a child's physical fitness level and body composition has less to do with genetics and more to do with learned behaviors, such as eating and exercise habits. Your children look up to you and learn from your actions. As a matter of fact, a recent study has shown that nearly 80 percent of kids inherit their fear of food, termed "neophobia," from their parents. These young neophobes often avoid healthy foods, like vegetables and whole grains, because they are unfamiliar with them, and the reason for this unfamiliarity is that their parents aren't eating them either. By adopting the principles you find in this book, you will also help your kids choose a healthy lifestyle.

You should read this book because it will help you work smarter. This book covers the principles behind fitness. As a result, you will discover how to create an overall fit lifestyle. Because you will know how to avoid the common pitfalls that can sabotage a fitness program, you will achieve fitness efficiently and effectively.

Finally, you should read this book to learn about how your body works and what you can do to make it run at its optimum. You'll learn the benefits of maintaining a regular fitness routine, plus strategies on how to follow through with your plans. You'll learn how to keep a positive attitude and avoid frustration and defeat. You'll learn how to maximize your body's potential through physical activity, healthy eating, hydration, and goal setting. This book will help you make your health and fitness a priority, so that you can enjoy a quality of life you never even imagined.

Understanding the Importance of Fitness

You only have one body and it has to last your whole life. Therefore, it is essential that you focus on fitness and make it a priority. By choosing to maintain and optimize your body's performance, you will experience an increase in health and vitality.

Being fit will give you more energy. You will be able to work hard all day and still have energy left over to play with your children or interact with your spouse and friends. Because you will be less tired at the end of the day, you will find that household chores that seemed overwhelming are now more manageable.

Another advantage of fitness is that you will sleep better. You will find it easier to achieve the kind of deep sleep your body needs to restore energy reserves and compensate for everyday wear and tear. As a result, you will awaken feeling refreshed and ready to start your day.

In large part, the lack of energy and functional losses we associate with aging are due to physical inactivity. A healthy, fit lifestyle will increase your vitality, helping you feel young and strong. As we age, it seems that we feel an inevitable loss of strength, energy, and stamina. However, this doesn't have to be the case. Those tasks that we dread becoming so difficult with aging, such as climbing stairs, carrying groceries, and walking to the mailbox, will be much easier throughout our lives if we remain physically active. When it comes to fitness, the old saying "use it or lose it" is true.

Finally, the good news is that it's never too late to get fit. Even a small amount of time invested in a weekly fitness routine can produce great health benefits. Spending just 30 minutes in moderate activity most days of the week can produce wonderful health benefits, including managing and preventing chronic illnesses from heart disease and diabetes to colon cancer and high blood pressure.

What are we doing wrong?

We have more responsibilities and less time to fulfill them than ever before. While we become busier every day, modern technology, such as personal computers, has decreased our amount of daily physical activity. As a result, recent studies have shown that more than 60 percent of adults in the U.S. do not get the recommended amount of exercise each day.

Our hectic, fast-paced lifestyle has also encouraged an increased dependence on fast food. An unhealthy diet, combined with a more sedentary lifestyle, has left Americans overweight and out of shape. Our poor fitness and dietary habits have led to America becoming the most obese country in the world. In fact, we are in the midst of an obesity epidemic that has led to a rise in preventable diseases like type-2 diabetes and cardiovascular disease. Some experts believe that as a result of obesity-related illnesses, Americans' life expectancy will soon begin to fall.

Our increasingly sedentary lifestyle is affecting us not just as individuals but on a national level. Studies have shown that those with an inactive lifestyle take more sick days and are less productive at work. Productivity declines are serious enough that many large companies have begun to include mandatory fitness regimens for employees. Studies have shown that employees who engage in even a bare minimum of physical activity during work show increased productivity, sense of purpose, and fulfillment with their jobs.

Many of us are under chronic job stress, which has been linked to heart disease and type-2 diabetes, as well as high blood pressure, insulin resistance, and excessive abdominal fat. Of course, it is possible to reverse many of the negative effects of stress with a few lifestyle changes.

On the whole, Americans eat more fat, sugar, and artificial sweeteners than any other country. The problem with the types of fats we eat is that the human body is nearly incapable of burning them. While we wait for energy from these fats, we grab something sweet for quick energy. It becomes a vicious cycle of fat and sugar, and we're left lethargic and depressed, with more fat being stored on our hips and around our middles.

Americans' poor eating habits, combined with the fact that we are less physically active than other nations, is leading us to become one of the most unfit countries in the world.

What are the solutions?

Unfortunately, there is no miracle pill or magic tonic that you can take to make you physically fit. With hard work and dedication, though, you can improve your fitness, mental outlook, and overall quality of life. Making fitness a priority in your life is the first step in the process of attaining a healthier life. Follow the principles in this book to learn how to incorporate fitness into your everyday life.

The good news is that you can control the condition of your body. By educating yourself about proper nutrition and healthy eating, along with getting the proper amount of exercise, you can improve your body. When you make healthier choices, like taking the stairs instead of the elevator or going to the gym instead of watching television, you can improve your overall physical fitness.

Change is possible, but it is up to you to take the first step. Cutting down on saturated, hydrogenated, and polyunsaturated fats, as well as sugars and artificial sweeteners, does work. The trick is to find healthy alternatives to your favorite foods. Healthy eating plus regular, moderate exercise is the key to unlocking your body's potential, improving your appearance, and enhancing your physical and mental health.

Maximizing the Benefits of This Book

Keep this book handy. Take it with you to work, to the gym, and to lunch with your friends. Refer to it often as you build a healthier, more fit, and happier you. The principles in this book will take time, commitment, and effort to realize. Read this book again and again as you make lifelong changes to your health and fitness.

This book is not an instructional manual on how to build a better body. Instead, it is a guide to building a healthier lifestyle. As you read this book, you will discover that fitness lies in changing yourself both mentally and physically.

Unlike some get-fit-fast or crash-diet schemes, this book relies on tested principles and significant research that will alter your perception of fitness before you even begin to work out. This book focuses on both mind and body as a guide to attainable and sustainable fitness goals.

You will get the best results if you read through this book and then reference it throughout the duration of your fitness regimen. While the principles contained here are presented in a straightforward manner, only by constantly reviewing the book will these principles become ingrained in you. This constant reinforcement will help you maintain your fitness regimen.

After you finish reading this book, leave it out and refer to it often so that your fitness discipline and eating strategies remain constant. When you have a question about your health, diet, or fitness, it will give you resources and direction to find the answers that are right for you.

Enjoy your life of health and fitness, and remember the wise words of American journalist and radio personality Franklin P. Adams: "Health is the thing that makes you feel that now is the best time of the year."

Benefiting from Fitness

Physical fitness will significantly improve your life, and perhaps even lengthen it. Not just for athletes and movie stars, and irregardless of age, capabilities, or gender, exercise has been shown to prevent chronic health conditions, boost self-confidence, esteem, and mood, and increase quality of life. Maintain a regular physical fitness routine and you will enjoy increased energy, a better overall mood, and greater physical and mental capacities.

Studies show that regular exercise has many benefits to your health, including preventing or managing such chronic health conditions as high blood pressure, high cholesterol, and type-2 diabetes. Another benefit of regular exercise is a stronger heart and lungs. As a matter of fact, individuals who exercise regularly improve their entire cardiovascular system—the circulation of blood through the heart and blood vessels. This means you'll have lots of energy to do the things you love.

While it may be obvious that working out regularly will result in physical changes, the changes in your mental outlook and mood could be even more significant. Because exercise stimulates the "happy" chemicals in your brain, you'll feel better, happier, and more relaxed, after just your first workout.

You will also notice a decrease in your anxiety, depression, and stress levels as you partake in regular exercise. If you have difficulty falling asleep, a daily physical routine will help.

Unfortunately, you can't get fit overnight. Remember, this is a lifestyle change. Fitness requires discipline, patience, and dedication. Allow yourself the time for your body to make significant changes. Do not become frustrated if you do not see immediate results. Remain determined and you will see the benefits and improvements.

The following principles emphasize the many benefits of physical fitness, the importance of individual progression, and the effort you can take to enjoy a healthier way of life.

Principle #1

Be active and live longer.

A U.S. Surgeon General's report on the benefits of physical activity concludes that moderate, regular exercise can substantially reduce the risk of developing diabetes, colon cancer, and obesity-related illnesses. Even a minimum of physical exercise increases the blood flow to all your major organs and throughout your body. As a result, you will be less prone to disease because toxins will have less opportunity to build up in your tissues. You will also be less prone to obesity because you will burn calories through activity that would otherwise be stored as fat. In this way, a healthy lifestyle that includes regular physical exercise will help you live a longer, healthier life.

PRINCIPLE #2

Counteract the effects of aging with physical activity.

There are few issues that so positively impact aging as physical activity. Regular physical activity helps build strong, healthy bodies and fights against particular diseases and ailments that are most associated with aging. Studies have shown that those who exercise regularly have a decreased chance of developing arthritis or osteoporosis. Exercising strengthens your muscles and increases bone density. While increased strength will improve your sense of balance, making you less apt to fall, increased bone density will help prevent fractures even if you do experience a fall. This means that you will maintain mobility even as you get older.

Principle #3

Exercise to decrease your risk of heart disease.

According to the American Heart Association, about 62 million Americans have some form of heart disease, killing 1 person every 34 seconds. Heart disease includes coronary heart disease, cardiovascular disease, high blood pressure, and heart failure. Many cases of heart disease could be prevented with regular exercise. Studies have shown that those who do not maintain a regular fitness routine more than double their risk of developing heart disease in their lifetime. Exercise strengthens the heart muscle and helps reduce cholesterol in the blood, which contributes to heart disease, so exercise daily to combat heart disease.

Principle #4

Increase lean muscle mass to burn more fat.

Muscle is the most effective fat-burning tissue in your body, so by increasing your lean muscle mass you accelerate your body's ability to burn fat. Because muscle tissue consumes calories both while your muscles are active and while they're at rest, the more muscle you have, the more calories you burn. As a matter of fact, studies have shown that for every pound of muscle you add to your body, you will burn an additional 35 to 50 calories per day. That means adding 10 pounds of muscle will burn up to 350 to 500 calories per day or 1 whole pound of fat every 7 to 10 days.

PRINCIPLE #5

Tone your muscles for a trim, athletic appearance.

Tone your muscles with exercise and enjoy a lean, firm physique as opposed to a flabby, saggy shape. Muscles that are repeatedly exerted at or near full capacity are forced to grow stronger in order to more effectively accomplish this new physical demand. Not only will your muscles grow stronger with exercise, but they'll also grow larger and more defined. Regular exercise, therefore, coupled with a decrease in body fat, which is the natural result of burning calories, will tone your muscles. As a result, your body will appear stronger, trimmer, and more athletic.

Principle #6

Improve and maximize your metabolism with regular exercise.

Metabolism is the process by which your body converts the food you eat into energy. In your body's cells, metabolism powers all your daily activities, from bike riding to reading to driving. Exercising improves your metabolism in 2 ways: first, it strengthens your heart's ability to pump blood, which carries nutrients and oxygen throughout the body. Second, your body responds to the demands for energy by speeding up its metabolism of food. This effect continues while you are at rest for 4 to 8 hours after exercising. The overall effect of being physically active on a regular basis, then, is to help you burn more calories, no matter what you're doing.

Principle #7

Enjoy more consistent and restful sleep when you exercise.

Your body alternates between states of activity and inactivity. It needs these 2 states to be in balance to maintain optimum performance. Studies have shown that if the body remains too sedentary during its active phase, it may have a difficult transition into sleep. However, by forcing your body to intensify its activity through exercise, you will allow it to enter into a deeper sleep during its period of inactivity. While you are awake, this increased and deeper sleep will enhance your vitality, mental acuity, and mood.

Principle #8

Exercise to decrease depression and anxiety.

Recently, promising research indicates that exercise helps some patients suffering from depression and anxiety feel better, even without medication. The research suggests that exercising 30 minutes a day, 3 to 5 days a week, can significantly improve the symptoms of depression. For those having difficulty getting started, even small bursts of activity, as little as 10 to 15 minutes at a time, can be a short-term mood enhancer. This is because exercise increases the brain's ability to produce endorphins, chemicals that relax muscles and give you an overall feeling of contentment. Those who regularly exercise report an increase in self-esteem and overall happiness.

PRINCIPLE #9

Enjoy newfound self-confidence.

As you begin to see and feel the results of your regular fitness routine, you will become more confident about your ability to accomplish the goals you set for yourself. As your hard work and dedication transform your body, and you feel stronger, leaner, and more physically fit, you will feel a sense of accomplishment and success. The realization that you are capable of sticking to a fitness plan and meeting your goals often has a collateral effect in the form of greater self-esteem, which will help improve other aspects of your life, such as your professional and social life.

Principle #10

Exercise to improve your social life.

People with sedentary lifestyles often find themselves isolated and lonely. By contrast, a healthy, active lifestyle is filled with opportunities for social interactions. For instance, find yourself surrounded with active individuals when you go for a nightly walk in your local park or take an exercise class at the gym. When you become more active you are likely to make friends who share your interest in exercise and fitness. With your newfound self-confidence, you are also more likely to strike up a conversation with fellow exercisers and pursue new opportunities for socializing. This will result in an improvement in your overall quality of life.

Principle #11

Enjoy fewer sick days with regular exercise.

Research shows that those who regularly exercise are less likely to get sick. During vigorous activity and exercise, your blood pressure increases, so the white blood cells and other immunity-boosting cells in your blood circulate through your body more quickly. This increased circulation allows for these cells to more efficiently kill bacteria and viruses, meaning you are less likely to get sick. Studies have also shown that those who participate in regular fitness routines take, on average, 40 to 50 percent fewer sick days from work. This is great news for you, and your boss!

PRINCIPLE #12

Enjoy social interactions while you exercise.

Remember when you were a child and exercise came in the form of hide-and-seek, hopscotch, or tether ball at recess. Exercise had a social element that kept you motivated and excited. Now, social interactions through exercise might be a casual conversation with someone while on the treadmill at the gym or an organized class or sport, such as spinning, yoga, or basketball. These social interactions will help you maintain a positive attitude toward working out, making it easier for you to stick with your fitness plan. In addition, socializing while you exercise makes you less likely to leave early or not go at all, because you're having so much fun.

PRINCIPLE #13

Exercise to help you quit smoking.

Studies show that light exercise, such as an evening stroll, can help reduce cigarette cravings and withdrawal symptoms. Scientists studying nicotine addiction have found that even a short 5-minute workout session can reduce a smoker's cravings for a cigarette. In addition to helping prevent weight gain, a benefit of exercise to smokers is fewer withdrawal symptoms, such as irritability, stress, anxiety, restlessness, tension, and poor concentration. Physical activity helps reduce the negative effects of cigarette withdrawal for up to 50 minutes after exercise. Studies also report that the desire to light up can be delayed 2 or 3 times longer than for those who do not exercise.

Principle #14

Improve brain function with walking.

—————————— ❋ ——————————

Have you ever taken a walk around the block when you are stuck on a problem at work? When you return, your head is clearer and you can think through the challenge much better. This is because when you exercise, it increases not only your blood circulation but also the oxygen and glucose that reach your brain. In effect, you are "clearing your head." When you partake in movement and exercise, you increase your breathing and heart rate. More blood flows to your brain, which enhances your energy production and waste removal. Essentially, you are oxygenating your brain—giving it just what it needs to function better.

Principle #15

Increase your cardiovascular fitness.

Cardiovascular fitness is simply how well your body is able to get oxygen and blood to its muscles. As your heart contracts, it pumps blood throughout your body. The number of times your heart contracts in a minute is your heart rate. The more rapidly your heart beats at its resting rate, or the harder it has to work to pump blood to your body, the less fit it is. You can improve your cardiovascular system's efficiency through regular cardio fitness training. During cardio exercise, your heart rate rises to meet your muscles' increased demand for oxygen. With regular exercise, your heart becomes more efficient and stronger.

PRINCIPLE #16

Lower your blood pressure with regular exercise.

Blood pressure is one of the principal vital signs of the human body. It is the force created by the circulation of blood on the walls of blood vessels as the heart pumps out blood. As your heart grows stronger in response to exercise, it can pump more blood with less force, and your blood pressure goes down. Studies have shown that those who maintain a regular workout routine and a reasonable body weight have a decreased risk of serious ailments such as high blood pressure, heart disease, and strokes.

Principle #17

Regulate and maintain proper body composition with regular exercise.

Body composition is the ratio of fat and lean (organs, bones, and muscle) tissues to the whole body's weight. You need the proper level of both muscle and fat for your body to function properly. For this reason, your body composition is an excellent gauge of your overall fitness. Too much fat is particularly harmful. Studies have shown that increased deposits of fat, especially around the mid-section, make you more susceptible to conditions such as diabetes, cardiovascular disease, and high blood pressure. Regular exercise regulates your body composition and improves your overall health.

Principle #18

Exercise to decrease body fat.

The consequences of too much body fat include increased risk of heart disease, stroke, diabetes, and even decreased immune function. This is why it is so important to control the fat that builds up when you take in more calories than your body needs. You will recognize this excess fat quickly as it often gathers around the waist, producing what is called a "spare tire." Some body fat is essential for good health, however, as it helps regulate body temperature, store energy, and insulates internal organs. Studies reveal a wide range of healthy percentages of body fat from about 5 to 25 percent for men and from 10 to 32 percent for women. A regular fitness routine, along with a proper diet, will decrease excess body fat.

Principle #19

Benefit from an exercise program, even if you have already lost weight.

Even if you have already reached your desired weight goal without exercising, your body will benefit from regular exercise. A thin person's body composition may have a high fat percentage and therefore be unhealthy. In particular, those who have undergone crash or extreme diets are particularly at risk of being unhealthy. Extreme diets can cause a loss of muscle mass instead of fat and can leave individuals vulnerable to the kinds of problems that afflict someone whose body composition consists of a high percentage of fat. On the other hand, regular exercise develops and maintains lean muscle while decreasing the body's percentage of fat.

Practicing the Keys to Success

There are, in essence, 4 keys to creating and maintaining a successful fitness routine. Together these keys to success will lay the foundation that will help you change your life and build a stronger, healthier, and more physically fit body. The keys to success are:

1. Set realistic goals
2. Create a plan
3. Keep track of progress
4. Celebrate achievement

These keys help ensure success by focusing on the positive aspects of working out. They help overcome the difficult mental obstacles that are common to any fitness program and focus on individual achievement, resulting in a routine that is easier to follow and more likely to be maintained. When you see evidence of your progress, you are more likely to maintain your efforts toward your personal fitness goals.

Often you will begin a fitness program with high hopes. Setting realistic goals will help maintain this excitement, even when you don't see immediate results or when you hit a plateau.

Creating a plan for your exercise program and having a routine in place can be the deciding factor on days you just don't want to work out. You'll likely have the extra little push you need on days when you are feeling sluggish.

Maintaining a record of your achievements can help you avoid creating a negative attitude toward physical activity. Try not to become frustrated if you miss a session or fail to reach a goal. Redirect yourself by imagining how you will avoid similar problems in the future. Remember that an occasional missed session is insignificant in the context of a new lifestyle that includes regular exercise.

The keys to success focus on using discipline and reinforcement in order to maintain a fitness routine, and they will help you shift your view of fitness to a way of life rather than simply a destination. The principles that follow will help you improve your body and mind by teaching you the keys to success.

Principle #20

Set realistic, challenging goals.

It's easy to become excited and overly ambitious when we begin a new fitness plan. Our newfound passion and motivation overwhelms our reason and we expect to run a marathon in 2 weeks when we've just begun our exercise program. When we fail to reach the lofty goal we've set for ourselves, we can become frustrated and quit. As a matter of fact, studies report that 50 percent of all people who start an exercise program quit within just a few short months. To avoid this pitfall, set goals that are difficult, but achievable. You should be challenged, but you should have opportunities for success. When you achieve a goal, you'll be proud of what you've accomplished and ready for the next challenge.

Principle #21

Build up to your goals.

You shouldn't expect to transform your body overnight but, rather, over a long period of time through hard work. Often those who try to make dramatic advances end up injuring themselves and stunting their long-term progress. Allow yourself time to make lasting advances. Establish a workout routine that first focuses on form and technique. Once your body has adapted to your new regimen, slowly intensify your workout. Building slowly toward your goals will help you reach your full potential. Regardless of your fitness goals, make exercise part of your daily routine and you will surely enjoy a longer, healthier life.

PRINCIPLE #22

Set short-, mid-, and long-term goals.

Every workout plan should contain short-, mid-, and long-term goals that both motivate you and allow you to measure your success. For instance, you might choose to run a 5K race in 4 months as your long-term goal. To prepare for the race, your short-term goal might be to walk or jog 2 kilometers without stopping. Your mid-term goals are the incremental goals you set for yourself. For instance, you might increase your walk or jog to 3 kilometers and then 4 kilometers during your training period. Determine your current level in all 3 fitness categories (cardiovascular, strength, and flexibility). You can set more realistic and achievable goals when you know what kind of shape you're in to begin with.

PRINCIPLE #23

Use visualization to improve results.

Before working out, visualize your routine. Imagine using proper form and accomplishing your workout goals. Studies have shown that people who prepare their minds and bodies through visualization are more likely to achieve their goals than those who do not prepare themselves. Visualize the specific aspects of the routine. If you are strength training, imagine the sounds the weights or the machine makes as you complete a repetition. If you are running, imagine the feeling of the road or treadmill under your feet. Visualize yourself achieving your goal and then go ahead and do it.

Principle #24

Take your time and avoid burnout.

Often, when we begin a new fitness regimen, we are eager for quick results. We push ourselves too hard, too soon. This push can result in burnout and/or injuring ourselves. You can't transform your body overnight, but you can injure yourself physically and mentally in no time. Remember to allow your body the time it needs to adapt properly to physical activity. Increase the intensity of your workouts only after you know your body is able to handle what you are currently asking of it. Adopt proper training methods to help assure that you will have beneficial and long-lasting results.

Principle #25

Don't expect changes to happen overnight.

It takes time for the body to change. Your body needs some time to adapt to your new fitness routine. You may even feel at first as though you're going in the wrong direction. Often people will gain weight or bulk when beginning a fitness routine due to the increase in muscle mass. Do not interpret this weight gain as failure, instead see this as the first tangible step to a healthier you. While some may see and feel differences more rapidly, you should allow between 6 and 8 weeks before you can see significant change. Then continue to measure your progress every 2 to 4 weeks.

Principle #26

Do not compare yourself to others.

Don't succumb to the pitfall of comparing your levels of fitness and accomplishment to those of others. Such comparisons can cause frustration and lead you to set unrealistic goals for yourself, which inevitably lead you to give up on your fitness program. Recognize that we all have different fitness potential and body composition, which lead to a variety of aptitudes and fitness levels. So, instead of measuring your success as it compares to others, measure it by the amount of effort you put forth, your attainment of your personal goals, and your body's physical improvements. Fitness is not about how you compare to others, but about motivating yourself to be as healthy as possible.

Principle #27

Plan your workouts ahead of time.

To maintain a serious fitness routine, you must make your workouts a priority. All too often we allow other aspects of our lives, such as work and family responsibilities, to derail our progress toward fitness. Skipping workout sessions because something "more important" comes up can quickly result in abandoning your fitness goals altogether. Block out time for your workouts on a calendar days or weeks in advance. Stick to your workout schedule in the same way you would keep any other important commitments. Make time for working out instead of working out if you have the time.

Principle #28

Make realistic changes to accommodate your workout program.

You should avoid attempting to make drastic changes in your life to accommodate a new workout program. Instead, look for opportunities to fit exercise into your existing lifestyle. For example, if you are not a morning person, it is probably unrealistic to plan to wake up and exercise before work, though this can be a great benefit to your metabolism. Instead, try working out in the early evening or even on your lunch hour. The right workout schedule is the one that you can and will stick to, so consider your lifestyle and personal preferences when scheduling your exercise.

Principle #29

Personalize your fitness routine by choosing activities you enjoy.

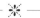

Working out shouldn't be work. It shouldn't be boring. And it shouldn't be the last thing you want to do every day. If you're not feeling motivated to workout, it's probably because your workouts aren't fun for you. Fitness plans work best if they incorporate your likes and dislikes. Examine your lifestyle and physical abilities: do you like dancing, bike riding, weight training, or snow skiing? If you choose activities that you enjoy and that stimulate you mentally and challenge you physically, you are going to be far more likely to stick with your fitness plan.

Principle #30

Diversify your workouts to avoid boredom and improve results.

Variety is the spice of life, and your fitness routine. Including an assortment of activities in your fitness routine will keep you from becoming bored and abandoning certain activities all together. For instance, mix up your cardio and strength-training regimen with a weekly Pilates class or a bike ride after work. Diversifying your workout will not only keep you from becoming bored, but it will also help you avoid injury. Repetitious workouts can lead to overworking certain muscles, which will result in strains and other injuries. You will enjoy and look forward to working out more when you add variety to your routine.

Principle #31

Maintain a positive attitude.

It is important to maintain a positive attitude toward your workout routine. And it is equally important to plan for days when you aren't feeling all that positive! Here are some things you can do to keep a positive attitude about your workouts: Make every effort to create workout sessions you look forward to. Avoid negative self-talk by replacing negative thoughts with positive thoughts. (For example, when you hear yourself think, "I'll never get in that bathing suit," change it to "My legs are getting toned with exercise.") Finally, don't let yourself become frustrated over a missed workout session. Instead, resolve to make sure you get to your next workout.

Principle #32

Start the day with exercise.

Starting your day with exercise is invigorating. When you exercise first thing, you prepare your body for the day by accelerating your circulatory system and getting much-needed oxygen to your muscles and your brain. Working out early in the day gives an extra boost to those looking to lose weight, since the body responds to exercise by increasing your metabolism. Your metabolism will remain at the higher level and thus you will continue to burn calories at a higher rate, even hours after you've worked out. Enjoy an early morning workout and feel the effects all day long!

Principle #33

Plan to work out with a partner, so you won't skip out.

A workout partner is a great motivator, especially when you've had a hard day and it is all too easy to find excuses to skip your workout. At times like these, it helps to have the extra pressure of knowing someone, besides yourself, is counting on you. Workout partners are a built-in backup plan to help you maintain your exercise schedule. It is important to pick a partner who has similar fitness goals and motivational level and who is eager to maintain a fitness routine. Some find it helpful to work out with a neighbor, roommate, or coworker; if your partner is someone you see on a regular basis, you are more likely to stay committed.

Principle #34

Replace self-doubt
with positive thoughts.

Henry Ford, founder of the Ford Motor Company and father of the modern assembly line, once said, "If you think you can do a thing or think you can't do a thing, you're right." We all experience moments when we doubt our abilities. It is important to be prepared for these moments and to form strategies for dealing with self-doubt. An excellent way to combat self-doubt is to replace your negative thoughts with positive ones. Take the time to write down a few of your fitness doubts and then create a positive redirection. For instance, "I can't swim a mile," becomes "I can swim a mile because I've been conditioning myself to do it."

Principle #35

Track your progress to maintain your focus.

Regularly monitor your progress to reinforce your effort and motivate you to reach your goals. You can track your physical accomplishments on the calendar you use for your workout schedule. Take note of your successes by placing a mark or star on the calendar. You will receive inspiration every time you look at it. Another approach is to place reminders of your goals around the house and office where you know you will see them every day. This constant visual reinforcement will help maintain focus on your goals.

Principle #36

Measure your weight accurately.

Your weight fluctuates throughout the day. You weigh the least when you first wake up, because your body has had all night to process food and water. By the end of the day you are heavier, because you are carrying all the food and water that you have consumed throughout the day and not yet processed. To get a more accurate measurement, weigh yourself as soon as you wake up in the morning. Weigh yourself without clothes and record your weight in a journal. You will be less likely to take that extra serving at dinner if you know that the effects of overeating will show up the next morning and be documented in black and white.

Principle #37

Use visual aids to set goals, motivate, and show success.

Create a system that will help you keep sight of your goals and measure your progress. When you keep records of your target goals, exercise frequency, and achievements, you will be more likely to stick with your routine. Even something as simple as a calendar with check marks or smiley faces on the days you worked out can help motivate you to exercise regularly. You will be better able to track your progress and see the results of your efforts if you record the type and intensity of your workouts. Seeing the progress you have made will motivate you to continue working out.

Principle #38

Measure your success according to your personal standards.

Each one of us has a different level of potential, which depends on many factors, such as our current level of fitness, our health, and our past experiences with physical activity. These factors should be kept in mind when setting goals and measuring progress. Avoid comparing yourself to others when you judge your successes. Instead, focus on the improvements you feel to your own physical and mental state. Before beginning your fitness program, establish a baseline level of fitness, focusing on your cardiovascular health, body composition, strength, and flexibility, and set goals tailored to your specific situation, not someone else's.

Principle #39

Maintain your focus to improve results.

Studies have shown that when working out, a strong level of focus helps improve results and minimize injuries. The reason for this is that if you are focused on the exercise you are doing, you are more likely to maintain proper form. With proper form, you will target the right muscles and are more likely to achieve the desired effect. Try not to be distracted by thoughts of what might be happening at work or at home. Remember that the world is unlikely to come to an end because you're taking a fitness break. Indeed, chances are good that you will return to your everyday duties refreshed and with new ideas and energy.

Principle #40

Celebrate your achievements.

Research shows that for a behavior change to become permanent, it needs to be reinforced properly. Giving yourself a reward for accomplishing your short-term goals will help you achieve long-term goals by maintaining focus and motivation. Reward yourself for both short- and long-term goals. Establish the reward in advance. Rewards, if possible, should be in keeping with your new, healthy lifestyle. If you are rewarding yourself for losing 10 pounds, for example, don't celebrate with a high-calorie meal. A more appropriate reward might be a new article of clothing that fits your slimmed-down figure. The right kind of reward can motivate you to continue your exercise routine in order to make further progress.

Principle #41

Build your self-confidence by noting success.

Every time you work out, you should take a moment to recognize that you have completed a task that you have set for yourself. These realizations will reinforce your confidence and help motivate you to continue working out. Every completed fitness routine proves that you can achieve what you put your mind to. Recall this realization when you get tired or bored with working out. It will boost your motivation and self-confidence. Realizing that you have achieved your objectives in the past will encourage you to continue to do so.

PRINCIPLE #42

Transfer your newfound confidence to other aspects of your life.

Studies show that exercise boosts the spirit and helps us feel good about ourselves. Enjoy the new confidence you feel in your improved physical appearance and bask in the realization that you are attaining your fitness goals. Know that if you can stick to your exercise program, you can successfully undertake improvements in other aspects of your life. Your new, positive outlook may give you the confidence you need to try new, exciting activities, and to pursue work and social endeavors that you were previously reluctant to try. Enjoy the world as it opens up to the new you!

Benefiting from Cardiovascular Training

Every fitness program should consist of 3 training components: cardiovascular, strength, and flexibility. No matter your body and fitness goals, it is important to include all 3 components in order to maximize your body's potential, minimize risk of injury, and avoid burnout. Training in each component enhances training in the others, resulting in optimal performance and better overall physical fitness.

The first component, cardiovascular training, involves repetitive exercises that require the heart and lungs to constantly replenish the muscles with oxygen and blood flow. For optimal cardio training, it is important to calculate your maximum heart rate and target heart rate. When you perform in the target range—60 to 80 percent of your maximum heart rate—your training will be the most effective. This chapter will show you how to calculate these figures.

Cardio training has many benefits for your health. As you vary the duration and intensity of your workouts, your heart responds to the need to work harder by growing stronger. As the heart gets stronger, your blood pressure will be lower, reducing your risk of strokes, diabetes, and kidney problems.

Common forms of cardiovascular training are running, walking, swimming, aerobics, and bicycling. To get fit, you should engage in cardio training 3 to 5 days a week, for 20 to 40 minutes each session. Because the heart and body take time to grow stronger, start with 20 minutes and work your way up to a longer, more intense program. A good place to begin, if you are fairly new to fitness, is a low-intensity, long-duration workout, such as walking. Over time, with consistent cardio workouts, you will find an increase in your stamina, endurance, and energy.

The following principles will help you understand the benefits of cardiovascular training and determine how to optimize your workouts to achieve the best results.

Principle #43

Combine cardio, strength, and flexibility training in your fitness routine.

A good fitness program includes the "Big 3": cardiovascular training, strength training, and flexibility training. In order to get the most out of your fitness routine, it is essential to include all 3 components in your workout plan. Even though your fitness goals may differ from those of other people, including all 3 aspects of fitness is essential to making the most of your body's potential. Inclusion of all 3 elements helps minimize risk of injury, optimizes performance, and helps avoid boredom and burnout. In addition, training in each area enhances your training in the other areas, which results in better overall performance.

Principle #44

Improve your heart's ability to pump blood with cardiovascular training.

Cardiovascular training improves your heart's ability to pump blood and provide oxygen to your muscles and other tissues. When you perform repetitious acts with only brief moments of rest, your heart is forced to adapt and improve its ability to pump oxygen-rich blood throughout the body. Activities such as running, walking, swimming, and bicycling are all excellent for cardiovascular training. When coupled with proper nutrition and adequate rest, cardiovascular training helps you increase muscular endurance in addition to improving your cardiovascular performance.

Principle #45

Improve blood circulation and reduce strain on your heart.

During physical activity, your pulse quickens and you breathe more deeply, signifying that you are using your cardiovascular system. As you condition your cardiovascular system to regular exercise, you are improving your blood circulation, which in turn reduces strain on the heart and prevents blood clots that can lead to heart attack and stroke. If you've had a heart attack, research has shown that regular physical activity can speed recovery, prevent the worsening of symptoms if you have heart disease, and reduce high-risk factors such as high blood pressure.

Principle #46

Increase blood flow and promote overall health with cardio.

Studies show that those who undergo regular cardiovascular training are experiencing physical benefits beyond those related to the heart and other muscles. Through cardiovascular training, your heart will become more efficient at pumping blood to the muscles and to all major organs. This improvement in the blood flow to major organs promotes better overall health, since proper organ function depends on an adequate blood supply. Increased blood flow also helps your muscles function better by making more oxygen available to them.

Principle #47

Protect bone mass through regular aerobic exercise.

Regularly engaging in aerobic exercise and cardiovascular training protects your body during weight loss and promotes healthy long-term gains. Those who undergo crash diets, fasting, and other forms of extreme weight loss often suffer from decreases in lean muscle mass and bone density. Often, the weight being lost is muscle and bone, not excess body fat. However, recent studies have shown that those who maintain regular cardiovascular training can eliminate this loss of lean muscle mass and bone density. In some cases individuals even increase bone density, therefore decreasing the risk of osteoporosis.

Principle #48

Elevate your mood and reduce stress through cardiovascular exercise.

Studies have shown that those who maintain a regular fitness routine that includes cardiovascular training enjoy a significant reduction of stress and increased mood elevation. Cardiovascular training has been shown to help stimulate the production of endorphins, which are naturally occurring chemicals associated with elevated mood and stress reduction. When you exercise, your body's ability to produce these chemicals is improved. Therefore the more you work out the better you feel, and the better you feel the more you work out. Thus, you begin a beneficial cycle of physical fitness.

PRINCIPLE #49

Choose cardiovascular activities that suit your needs.

Before selecting a cardiovascular activity, it is important that you consider your personal preferences and the condition of your body. Cardiovascular training varies in its degree of impact, level of intensity, and duration of exercise, so the current condition of your body will be a significant determining factor in choosing the proper cardiovascular training for you. For example, if you suffer from lower back or joint pain, you should choose activities, such as swimming or walking, that are relatively low-impact. It is important to select an activity that fits your circumstances so that you can stick to it.

Principle #50

Determine which low- or high-impact activities are beneficial for you.

Impact refers to the amount of force an activity exerts on the body. Activities that are considered high-impact, like running and kickboxing, require your body to absorb the full force of your weight hitting. These are excellent forms of exercise that can be done anywhere, with little specialized equipment. However, high-impact activities may not be appropriate for those with back, foot, or knee problems, or other joint ailments. Low-impact activities like swimming, bicycling, and walking are an excellent alternative to these high-impact exercises, and are equally beneficial. Know your limitations and select an appropriate activity for your specific circumstances.

Principle #51

Use the Talk Test to determine your cardio workout intensity.

A common mistake that people make is not measuring the intensity of their workouts. Intensity is the amount of energy that you use when you exercise. Your cardio workouts should not be so challenging that you burn out. Nor should they be so easy that you find yourself frustrated by a lack of results. A simple, accurate way to gauge your workout intensity is to take the Talk Test. The goal is to work out at a level at which you can answer questions, but not carry on a conversation. If you have to breathe between each word you say, you are probably working too hard. If you can sing your favorite song, you are probably not working hard enough.

Principle #52

Maintain intensity throughout your routine for optimum results.

Studies have shown that to achieve the maximum results, you should do cardio for at least 30 minutes a day, 3 times a week. In addition, to get the best results from your training, it is important that you maintain a steady level of intensity throughout each session. Therefore, you must select an exercise with a level of intensity that you can sustain throughout the duration of your workout. Maintaining a steady intensity throughout the duration of your 30-minute session will help you get the most from your workout.

Principle #53

Know your maximum heart rate to improve your workout efficiency.

The most accurate way to measure your workout intensity is to know your target heart rate (THR). Your THR is based on your maximum heart rate (MHR) and it is an estimate of where your heart rate should be when you are training aerobically. Maximum heart rate is the estimated number of beats per minute your heart is capable of producing and is directly related to your age. To determine your MHR, subtract your age from 220. For example, a 40-year-old would have an MHR of 180. Next, your THR zone is 60 to 80 percent of your MHR, or 108 to 144 beats per minute for the example. If you are working within this zone, you will improve your workout efficiency.

Principle #54

Use your target heart rate to train for specific fitness goals.

Once you know your maximum heart rate and target heart rates, you can train for specific fitness goals. For example, if want to improve your muscular endurance, you should attempt to raise your heart rate between 60 and 70 percent of your maximum heart rate. To improve your aerobic conditioning, you should train between 70 and 80 percent of your maximum heart rate. By training within these specific zones, you can target specific aspects of your cardiovascular health.

PRINCIPLE #55

Spend at least 20 minutes on aerobic exercise to begin to burn stored fat.

You must first burn through the calories your muscles and cardiovascular system have stored before your body begins to convert stored fat into energy. It typically takes 20 minutes of steady aerobic exercise before your body begins to draw on its fat supply. If you are looking to effectively lose weight, you should maintain an exercise program that focuses on low-intensity exercise for long durations. The longer you do your cardio exercises, the more stored fat your body will be forced to convert into energy.

Principle #56

Proceed with caution when recovering from an injury.

Even a minor injury can be made much worse if you go back to your customary cardio workout routine too soon. Consult your doctor about the best exercises for strengthening the injured part of your body. Your doctor may suggest a series of exercises or refer you to a physical therapist for the rehabilitation. It's important when recovering from an injury to take your time. Be very cautious and focus on flexibility training and low-intensity strength training as you make your way back to fitness. As you become stronger, duration and intensity should be gradually increased.

Principle #57

Even if you are looking to gain weight, don't ignore cardiovascular training.

Cardiovascular training is very important, even if you are looking to gain weight. Cardio training is critical for keeping your heart in good shape, which means it is a significant factor of your overall health. Include two 20-minute, low-intensity cardiovascular training sessions each week along with your regular strength-training activities. This limited cardiovascular training will not lead to weight loss, but it will ensure that you receive the many benefits of cardiovascular workouts, such as a stronger heart and increased blood flow to your muscles.

Principle #58

Engage in aerobic exercise for 20 to 40 minutes 3 times a week.

Studies show that in order to receive the maximum results from cardiovascular training, it is important to engage in aerobic exercise for 20 to 40 minutes at least 3 times a week. When first beginning a program, you should allow for at least 1 day of rest between these aerobic workout sessions. This provides your body with sufficient time to rest and repair itself. Over time, as you get in better shape, you can decrease the amount of rest days you take and intensify your cardiovascular training to achieve the maximum benefits from your cardio routine.

Principle #59

Choose high-intensity cardio to burn calories and low-intensity to burn fat.

Both low- and high-intensity training will help strengthen your body, improve your mood, stave off chronic illness, and lessen the effects of aging. The best type of cardio exercise for you depends on your fitness level and workout goals. For instance, if your goal is to lose weight, and your body can handle it, high-intensity activities burn calories faster and crank up your metabolism, so you continue to burn calories after exercise. If your goal is to tone and strengthen, low-intensity activities, such as walking, swimming, and elliptical machines, may be the better choice, as these activities burn more fat over longer periods of time and are less stressful on the body.

Principle #60

Vary your cardiovascular activities so you don't plateau.

Your body grows stronger when it is forced to adapt to new degrees of force. When you constantly expose your body to the same force or to just one certain exercise, your performance quickly plateaus. In order to avoid performance plateau and get rid of workout boredom, vary your cardiovascular exercises. Your body will respond by growing stronger when it is forced to work in new ways and you will find that switching your routine will invigorate you. This variety also allows for you to target different areas of the body while improving your overall cardiovascular health.

Getting Fit with Strength Training

The second component of your fitness plan will be strength training. This type of training focuses on the systematic overloading of your skeletal muscles in order to increase your body's ability to perform work.

Strength is measured by the amount of force your muscles can produce. Strength training is an anaerobic exercise, which means that your muscles do not consume oxygen as they work. Strength training involves explosive activities, like weight lifting or sprinting, that target and activate specific muscles near or at their maximum output for a short period or burst. By forcing your muscles to adapt to higher levels of resistance through activities like weight training, they will grow stronger and be better able to respond to sudden demands.

Your strength-training workouts will vary in intensity based on the number of sets and repetitions, the weight lifted, and the rest you give yourself between sets. It is recommended to practice 8 to 12 repetitions of 8 to 10 exercises, at a moderate intensity, 2 days a week; however, your program will vary based on your fitness goals. For instance, one person may be looking to build lean muscle and definition, another person may be interested in building muscle mass and increasing strength, and someone else may want to strength train to lower bad cholesterol.

As with all 3 components of training, you will need to gradually build up to an optimal strength-training program. Your body will indicate the level you are ready for. It is important to always use proper form and exercise caution during strength training to avoid injury.

As this chapter indicates, there are many benefits of strength training, including a reduction in stress, depression, and muscle and bone loss. Use the following principles to create an effective strength-training program and enjoy the health benefits of your new, fit lifestyle.

Principle #61

Boost your overall health with strength training.

A regular strength-training routine will increase your lean muscle mass, increase your metabolism, and help you prevent injury. Recently it has been reported that strength training may improve the way your body processes sugar, which may reduce the risk of developing diabetes. More benefits of strength training include stronger bones, weight management, reduced risk of injuries, increased energy and stamina, improved body image, and lower incidence of insomnia. Increased muscle fitness resulting from strength training also helps improve balance, mobility, and muscular endurance, and improves your body's form and posture.

Principle #62

Combine your cardio and strength training into one workout session.

Combining cardio and strength activities is a balancing act worth the work. Though you need both aerobic and strength training for optimum health, it's best to follow your strength training with cardio for a more effective workout. When cardiovascular training is done first, muscle fatigue severely diminishes your ability to weight train. However, by strength training first, you lower your blood sugar, which allows stored fat to be converted into energy during your cardiovascular training. Thus, the double session workout increases the amount of fat you burn and is more time-efficient.

PRINCIPLE #63

Balance your cardio to strength activity.

Of course you want to improve your health, body composition, and ultimately your appearance. To do so your workout program will need the right balance of strength to cardio activity. Often, men do minimal cardio and lots of weights; women tend toward the reverse, lots of cardio and no strength work. Everyone needs both! Cardio is essential to our long-term health and improved appearance; strength training decreases natural lean muscle tissue mass, shapes our muscles, and increases our basal metabolic rate. So, what's the right balance of cardio to strength work for optimal health, fitness, and weight management? Schedule 3 to 5 sessions of 30 minutes or more of cardio and 2 to 3 sessions of strength work per week.

PRINCIPLE #64

Overload your muscles to gain strength.

Strength training is the systematic overloading of your skeletal muscles in order to increase their strength and ability to work. Using resistance to contract muscles, strength training builds the size, strength, and anaerobic endurance of skeletal muscles. Strength training is an anaerobic (without air) exercise, working without the need of oxygen replenishing by the heart. Activities focus on displays of explosive strength and power (sprinting, weight lifting, etc.) by working targeted muscles at or near their maximum output for a short period. With the addition of periods of rest, your body will become stronger and more able to deal with these new requirements.

Principle #65

Create stronger tendons and ligaments with strength training.

Properly performed, strength training can result in significant functional benefits and overall health improvement. Your form and posture will become stronger with an increase of skeletal muscle. You will feel that your body functions and moves better. Strength training increases the strength and toughness of bones, muscles, tendons, and ligaments, making the body stronger and less susceptible to injury. Stronger muscles, tendons, and ligaments, along with improved posture, allow you to move with more fluidity, which will help you to avoid injuries.

Principle #66

Prevent loss of bone density
with strength training.

As we get older, a natural part of aging is the loss of bone density. Similarly, recent studies have shown that those who engage in rapid weight loss, through extreme diets for instance, often suffer from more severe decreases in bone density. This serious condition can affect an individual's overall health and contribute to osteoporosis. Include strength training in your weight-loss plan to avoid a loss in bone density. Some individuals even see signs of increases in their bone density. For those who already have osteoporosis, strength training can lessen its impact.

Principle #67

Increase your HDL and lower your LDL cholesterol with strength training.

Several studies confirm that the benefits of strength training include increasing our HDL, or "good" cholesterol levels, and lowering our LDL, or "bad" cholesterol levels. While cardiovascular training has long been known to help reduce the amount of harmful LDL cholesterol in the human body, recent studies have shown convincing links between strength training and increased HDL cholesterol in the body's arteries. Healthy cholesterol levels significantly lower your risk of heart disease and other related medical conditions and improve your overall cardiovascular health.

Principle #68

Alleviate symptoms of depression and reduce stress with strength training.

Studies have shown that strength training is associated with increased levels of dopamine, serotonin, and norepinephrine (it's been found that depletion in one or more of these neurotransmitters may cause mood disorders, including depression and bipolar disorder). Directly targeting the pleasure centers of the brain, exercise causes an increase of these chemicals, resulting in enhanced feelings of well-being and improving your self-esteem and self-confidence. Additionally, working out with strength training reduces the physical and biochemical causes for stress.

Principle #69

Counteract the process of "sarcopenia" with strength training.

Sarcopenia is the process of losing muscle as we age—a condition every one of us will experience in our lifetime. Each of us loses about ½ pound of muscle each year after the age of 30. This amounts to about 5 pounds by age 40, and with each decade, this process accelerates. In addition, this loss of muscle is nearly always replaced with fat, leading to an excess of body fat as we age. This process is slow, but steady and inevitable. Because of its ability to build and restore muscle mass and also to increase our metabolism, strength training is a natural antidote for sarcopenia.

Principle #70

Avoid using weight inertia to complete repetitions.

The term inertia describes movement energy. In other words, inertia is the force that opposes the change of movement velocity. When lifting weights, it is not enough to lift just the force of gravity acting upon the weight you are lifting. You have to use additional force to move the object. Once the object is moving, you have to use your muscles to control its speed. Finally, you have to use additional force to complete the repetition. When you use your muscles to control the movement of the weight all the way through the repetition, you avoid using inertia. As a result, your muscle gets stronger.

Principle #71

Choose weight, elastic, or hydraulic resistance.

Weight resistance is a common, effective form of resistance training where you use your muscle strength to complete each repetition. Elastic resistance relies on elastic bands to create tension as they are stretched. When the band is stretched, it results in an increase of resistance as the band is expands. Hydraulic resistance creates a constant force that works against the muscle uniformly during the entire repetition. These expensive resistance machines are usually found only in a gym. Mix and match to determine which option is most effective for you.

PRINCIPLE #72

Use isometric training to work specific points of your muscles.

Activating a muscle in a fixed position forces it to contract while the joint and muscle positions remain stable. Traditional forms of strength training rely on the lengthening and shortening of the muscles. Isometrics, on the other hand, train a specific point on the muscle. Caution should be taken, however, as isometric exercises may be hazardous to perform due to the large amount of weight and the static nature of the exercise. You should have a professional instruct you in isometric training before undertaking any strenuous exercises.

Principle #73

Use household items to strength train.

✳

A common misconception about strength training is that you'll have to join an expensive facility or buy a costly home gym with weight machines and dumbbells to have a successful training program. This just isn't true. If a gym membership or at-home weight-training equipment are not accessible to you, don't fret. Resistance training can be performed practically anywhere. All it takes is a little creativity. Use 1-gallon bottles of bleach, orange juice, or milk, and 1- and 5-pound bags of pasta, rice, or beans for arm training. Squat and lunge with a 10-pound bag of dog food for leg training. Household items can make very convenient weights, and it is fun to be creative.

Principle #74

Perfect your form for the best results.

Since strength training relies on the isolation and overloading of specific muscles, it is essential to learn proper technique. Without proper form, you will see little increase in strength and risk being injured. Frequently, we learn weight-training techniques by watching others at the gym; however, sometimes this leads to modeling incorrect technique. Using improper technique can result in chronic injuries, including rotator cuff damage, muscle overload, bone stress injuries, and nerve damage. It is recommended you make an appointment with a personal trainer before beginning any strength-training program. Professional, accredited trainers can help you perfect your form and personalize your strength-training program.

Principle #75

Exercise muscles in proper progression to maximize results.

An important element of strength-training exercise is sequence. If your workout includes a variety of weightlifting exercises, it is advisable to begin with your larger muscle groups and move to the smaller muscles. This allows for optimal performance of the most demanding exercises when your fatigue levels are at their lowest and you feel energized and fresh. The most important thing is to be sure that you have enough energy to complete your entire workout. It is better to do less and complete the entire circuit than to neglect a muscle group.

Principle #76

Increase your muscle mass by increasing weight and decreasing repetitions.

You can manipulate the amount of resistance, repetitions, and sets your strength-training sessions include to target specific goals. For instance, in order to increase your muscle mass and build large muscles, weight should be increased and the number of repetitions decreased. Allow for a slight increase in the amount of time you rest between sets. Remember when you are training for strength, the focus of your workout should be the increase of quick explosive strength. Lift at 80 to 90 percent of your maximum weight. Lifting heavy weights alone can be very dangerous, so have a partner or gym employee stand nearby, just in case you need assistance.

Principle #77

Decrease weight and increase repetitions for more muscle definition.

If your goal is to enhance your muscle tone and endurance, increase the amount of repetitions and decrease the resistance of your strength-training program. When you decrease the level of resistance and increase the amount of repetitions of your workout, you are training your muscles to work at an optimum level. You will see considerable advances in your muscle tone and strength, without seeing significant gain in the size or bulk of your muscles. If you want to create long, lean muscles, you should train at around 60 to 70 percent of maximum intensity for 15 to 20 repetitions each set.

Principle #78

Increase muscular endurance by decreasing rest time between sets.

Muscular endurance, the ability to sustain muscle contractions repeatedly before reaching the point of fatigue, is very important for playing sports or doing an activity for a long period of time. To increase muscular endurance with strength training, decrease your rest periods between sets. This will force your muscles to more rapidly prepare for work. Also, drop down to 40 to 60 percent of your maximum intensity and increase your repetitions to 20 or more. You can also increase muscular endurance by slowing the contraction of your muscles and increasing the length of time it takes you to lift.

Principle #79

Use your body weight to develop strength.

Our bodies are an amazing and often untapped source of resistance for strength training. We all know the typical bodyweight exercises, including pushups, sit-ups, pull-ups, and dips. These exercises are great for fitness and endurance training as they use the fixed resistance of our body weight. The key to strength training, however, is to increase the amount of resistance over time. The way to do this is to decrease the amount of leverage we exert on the exercise. For example, we can effectively double the difficulty of a hanging tucked leg lift by straightening our legs, thus building strength with just body weight.

Principle #80

Choose at least one strength-training exercise for each major muscle group.

To prevent injuries, strength-training routines should include at least 1 exercise for each of the major muscle groups: the gluteals (your rear-end), quadriceps (front thigh), hamstrings (back thigh), hip abductors and adductors (inner and outer thigh), calves (back lower leg), lower back, abdominals (stomach), pectoralis major (upper chest), rhomboids (upper back between shoulder blades), trapezius (upper back from neck to shoulder), latismus dorsi (mid-back), deltoids (cap of shoulder), biceps (front upper arm), and triceps (back upper arm). Be sure your weekly program includes exercises for each of these muscle groups to create a balanced workout.

Increasing Flexibility

It is common for flexibility training to get overshadowed by its counterparts, cardiovascular and strength training; however, flexibility training strengthens tendons and ligaments, resulting in improved muscle performance and reduced risk of injury.

Flexibility training is more than simply stretching before and after workouts (although that is an important component). This type of training involves manipulating your body's joints in order to increase your strength and range of motion. Flexibility training may consist of slow, fluid motions that target specific locations on a joint's range of motion, or it may consist of rapid, sweeping movements that target the joint's entire range of motion. Increasing your flexibility will enable you to make significant advances in your strength, endurance, and balance while decreasing your chances for injury.

Flexibility training involves many different types of stretching. You can practice isometric, static, resistance, or dynamic stretching techniques, all of which will benefit the rest of your fitness program. The principles in this chapter will teach you the benefits of each type of stretching and will explain the proper (and improper) ways to perform these exercises.

After incorporating flexibility exercises, you will quickly see the benefits in the other areas of your training. You will enjoy increased power during weight lifting, lessened muscle soreness after cardio workouts, fewer injuries, and a reduction in stress. Flexibility training is wonderful because it can be done practically anywhere, at any time, at any age. Practices like yoga can be enjoyable, effective ways to include flexibility training in your weekly workouts.

Use the principles in this chapter to perform a variety of flexibility exercises to complement your cardio and strength training. You will quickly see the myriad rewards in your fitness level and overall well-being.

Principle #81

Begin and end every workout session with stretching.

Every workout session should begin and end with flexibility training or stretching. Warm-up stretches before you exercise prepare the body for work by increasing blood flow to the muscles and by relieving tension in the muscles. Warming up before working out reduces the risk of injuries. After completing your workout, it is important to cool down with stretching. In this way, your body is allowed to gently unwind from the vigorous work it has just undergone. A proper cool down will also help reduce muscle soreness.

PRINCIPLE #82

Warm up first and hold your stretches.

Stretching is a great way to reduce anxiety and muscle tension, as well as lower your breathing rate and blood pressure. Though it can be an effective relaxation technique, it should always be preceded by a short 5- to 10-minute warm-up. Warm-ups like jogging in place, brisk walking, and stationary biking prepare your muscles, ligaments, and tendons for stretching. Holding the stretches is also essential as it increases the amount of blood flow to the joints' connective tissue. The more blood and oxygen the tissue receives, the better you will be able to perform under strain. Maintaining a stretch for at least 8 seconds forces the muscle to relax in its full-extended position. This loosens the muscle and makes it less susceptible to injury.

Principle #83

Improve muscle performance with flexibility training.

Stretching the joints of your body prior to strength and cardio training increases their range of motion and fitness for the workout ahead. Often overlooked, flexibility training is an essential factor in getting the most out of your body. When you target specific locations on a joint's range of motion through flexibility training, it helps increase the blood flow to your muscles, tendons, and ligaments. In other words, it warms up your body for the challenges to come. Use flexibility training to prepare your body for exercise. It will help you to maintain proper form, thus decreasing the likelihood of injury.

Principle #84

Use flexibility training to prevent injury.

Flexibility training helps prevent injury by improving the range of motion of your joints. By increasing circulation to muscles and connective tissues, stretching creates an increase in muscular elasticity. This allows your muscles to function better under extreme stress and thus you will achieve higher levels of performance without injury. Increased flexibility aligns your body by strengthening the tendons, ligaments, and muscles that maintain its shape or posture. Stronger tendons and ligaments protect your muscles and help prevent them from becoming strained or knotted.

Principle #85

Use passive stretching and deliberate breathing to target specific muscles.

An important form of stretching is called passive stretching, which utilizes deliberate breathing. This form of flexibility training focuses on the full extension of a joint to its maximum position and then holding that position for a period of time, usually about 30 seconds. During passive stretching, you should concentrate on slow and deliberate breathing, which will help relieve tension as you move further into each stretch. This form of stretching allows you to target specific muscle groups. With a partner's help or the help of an immovable prop, you can stretch your body to its apex and hold for up to 30 seconds.

PRINCIPLE #86

Use static stretching to become more flexible.

Through the manipulation of opposite muscle groups, a technique called static stretching, you can effectively increase a joint's range of motion. Used to stretch the muscles while the body is at rest, static stretching lessens the sensitivity of tension receptors, which allow your muscles to relax and be stretched to a greater length. During this type of flexibility training you slowly move toward the extreme position of a joint, holding the stretch for 10 to 13 seconds at the joint's apex. As your body relaxes, the joint will become more flexible. Over time, you will find that your joints loosen and allow for a better stretch and greater range of motion.

Principle #87

Engage your muscles while stretching to achieve greater flexibility.

Engaging your muscles during stretching will help lengthen them. Assuming a passive stretch position, stretch and tense the muscle for 7 to 15 seconds, then release and allow it to relax for at least 20 seconds. An example is folding in a forward bend, then tensing your hamstrings to achieve a greater stretch. Due to the strain placed on your ligaments, this type of stretching (known as isometric stretching) should be done only after your body is thoroughly warmed up. This form of stretching should be avoided by children and elderly individuals because of the increased strain placed on the body.

Principle #88

Use dynamic stretching to work the entire range of the joint.

Dynamic stretching exploits the full range of the joint. This form of stretching uses speed and momentum to achieve the stretch. Unlike other forms of stretching, dynamic stretching does not include holding a stretch. Rather it is a moving stretch. Examples of dynamic stretching include trunk twists and simulated kicking. This type of stretching is often used to improve the flexibility of specific joints as they are applied for specific sports. For instance, a tennis player may perform a mock serve without racket or ball.

PRINCIPLE #89

Use resistance stretching to lengthen muscles.

When you do resistance stretching, you rely on a partner to stretch your joint to its apex as you actively contract the opposing muscle. This form of flexibility training targets the entire range of motion of the joint and length of the muscle. Have your partner extend the joint slowly with a force only slightly stronger than that which you exert against them. Because of risk of injury, it is recommended that you receive expert instruction before engaging in this type of flexibility training.

Principle #90

Try yoga as a fun and effective method of flexibility training.

Yoga can be a fun and effective method of lengthening and strengthening muscles for greater flexibility. The myriad benefits of yoga—aside from improving flexibility markedly—include better posture, increased stamina, increased energy, improved balance, and injury prevention and recovery. Yoga classes are available at gyms and private studios and are offered for every age and skill level. To that point, a recent study from the American Council on Exercise concluded that yoga is "a valuable addition to any exercise routine, offering the essential elements of flexibility, balance and relaxation; factors often neglected in traditional workouts."

Principle #91

Gain muscle power for your workouts with flexibility training.

Flexibility training will give you added muscle power while it strengthens and lengthens your muscles. Muscle power refers to the load the muscle can move and how quickly it can move it (versus muscle strength, which refers to the size of the muscle mass, its ability to hold pressure, and the tension it can bear without tearing). Muscles have the most power when the individual muscle fibers are at their longest length of contraction. This is when the muscle can move a larger load more quickly. Therefore, by lengthening your muscle fibers through flexibility training, you gain power to aid your workout routine.

Principle #92

Consider external factors that may impede your flexibility training.

You may have existing conditions that impede your body's flexibility. These may include injury to the muscles and other connective tissue, degradation of muscles and tissue with age, your degree of body activity, the level of water within your body, and an excess of fatty tissue. Take all these factors into consideration when creating an effective flexibility-training program. For example, consider that certain exercises, such as squats, may be detrimental if you have a knee injury. Your goal is to improve your body without exposing it to further damage.

Principle #93

Focus on breathing for greater flexibility.

Proper breathing control can significantly impact your flexibility training. Your body naturally tenses up under the strain of stretching, resulting in you holding your breath. However, holding your breath decreases the range of motion and denies your joints oxygen. Concentrate on slow breathing. Allow your breathing to become regular before intensifying a stretch. Always extend a stretch during the exhaling portion of a breath. Slow, deliberate breaths while you are stretching increase your flexibility and ability to relax into the stretch, increasing blood flow throughout your body, and helping to remove lactic acid and other exercise by-products.

Principle #94

Avoid overstretching.

Just as your body can become weaker and injured by overexertion during strengthening and cardio training, it can become damaged from overstretching during flexibility training. Pay attention to your body as you stretch. You should experience mild discomfort, but no pain. Your body should not be sore the day after you have stretched. If you do feel pain, it is an indication that you are probably overstretching. Overstretching will increase the time it takes for you to gain more flexibility as your damaged muscles must repair themselves and will not offer the same flexibility until they have done so. Stretch only to the point that you feel strong resistance.

Principle #95

Avoid bouncing when stretching.

Bouncing during stretching, or ballistic stretching, can lead to serious injury and should be avoided. Examples of ballistic stretching include bending forward with your knees straight and bouncing while you reach for your toes. Avoid sudden jerking or accelerating during stretching. The sudden jarring movements can increase the chance of injury. Stretching motions should be fluid and without sudden acceleration or deceleration. If you are bouncing, it is very likely that you are overexerting yourself. Decrease the intensity to a point where you do not need to bounce in order to hold a position. For instance, it is better to bend your knees slightly to reach your toes, rather than bouncing.

Principle #96

Massage muscles to help them warm up for flexibility training.

Massaging a muscle prior to stretching or strength exercises for those muscle groups can be very beneficial and can improve performance. Massage increases blood flow and improves circulation; relaxes muscles; prevents painful cramps; and helps remove waste products, such as lactic acid, which prevents post-exercise soreness. Taking the time to massage muscles you're about to work out can make flexibility and strength exercises easier and more useful.

Eating a Healthy Diet

The food choices we make, how frequently we eat, and how much we eat all play a significant and defining role in the condition of our bodies. When we select low-calorie, high-nutrient foods that have little or no chemicals added to them, we give our bodies the high-quality fuel and organic material that helps maintain our health and fitness.

You will both look and feel better when you eat the right foods. Scientific studies have repeatedly found a strong connection between food and mood. Incorporating complex carbohydrates like fruits, vegetables, and whole grains into your diet helps maintain levels of scrotonin, a mood elevating chemical in the brain.

Healthy food choices also provide your body with the nutritional requirements it needs to function optimally without adding extra calories. Eating these kinds of foods in the form of smaller meals throughout the day provides energy and nutrition, raises our metabolism, and keeps us from having cravings. Poor nutritional value—found in such oft-consumed foods as junk food, soda, and refined sugars—strips the body of nutrients and piles on the calories. Chemical processing and hormone enrichment in many of the foods we eat are contributing to an overall decrease in health and quality of life for many Americans.

While there is a growing trend toward organic products, eating healthy doesn't have to mean eating organic foods only. For most people, the expense and limited availability makes this impossible at this time. You can choose, however, to eat foods that naturally occur in nature. These foods will be more easily broken down and processed by the body.

Many people make the mistake of overlooking the significant role of food choices when starting a fitness program. The following principles will educate you about healthy eating choices that will further enhance your new active lifestyle.

Principle #97

Consult the *Dietary Guidelines for Americans* to determine your needs.

Experts recommend using the *Dietary Guidelines for Americans* in order to ensure that your meals are nutritional and calorically balanced for your body's needs. The *Dietary Guidelines for Americans* are scientifically based determinations on ideal diets based on age, gender, and physical activity. They state not only the ideal about what an individual should eat but also how they should prepare the food and what level of activity they should maintain to be fit. Use the dietary guide to ascertain your proper nutrient requirements. For more information about the *Guidelines*, go to www.health.gov/DietaryGuidelines.

Principle #98

Follow the USDA Food Pyramid.

The secrets to eating right to get fit include finding a proper balance between food and physical activity, making the most out of the calories you consume, and staying within your daily calorie needs. The USDA has determined 6 food groups and how much should be eaten from each group for optimal nutrition. Experts suggest 6 to 11 servings from the grain group and 3 to 5 servings of vegetables. Enjoy 2 to 4 servings of fruit and 2 to 3 servings of dairy. The recommended 2 to 3 servings from the protein group should focus on lean meats, such as fish and chicken. Lastly, choose sparingly from the fats, oils, and sweets category. For personalized plans and interactive tools to help you plan your food choices, visit www.MyPyramid.gov.

PRINCIPLE #99

Practice portion control to conquer cravings.

Don't deny yourself your favorite foods. Instead, eat these foods in smaller portions or choose healthier options. Diets that force us to stop eating our favorite foods often lead to "cheating" or bingeing later. A good tip is to wait 20 minutes from the initial craving. If after 20 minutes you still crave the food, then go ahead and have some. If you eat a small amount slowly, enjoying every single bite, you can curb the craving. Or choose a healthier option, such as pretzels instead of potato chips when you find yourself wanting something crunchy and salty. Conquer your cravings by learning to control them.

Principle #100

Determine whether your food cravings are due to a lack of nutrients.

If you overindulge in sweet or salty food, it may be that your cravings are due to a lack of essential vitamins and minerals. For instance, if you crave chocolate, your diet may lack magnesium. Find magnesium in raw nuts, seeds, legumes, and fruits. If you crave sugar, your body may need chromium, among other things. Find chromium in broccoli, grapes, cheese, dried beans, calf liver, and chicken. Getting enough nutrients and minerals may help prevent cravings. However, even with your new, healthy diet, you will probably still have a few favorite foods that you like to enjoy, and it is important to allow yourself the occasional treat, in moderation.

Principle #101

Plan meals in advance to ensure a healthy and nutritionally balanced diet.

If you plan your meals in advance you will be less likely to be tempted by fast food, sugary snacks, and other unhealthy choices. We often make poor food choices and eat far more than we need to when we are very hungry. Try planning out your next meal just after eating or while you are still full from a previous meal. Or plan your meals a week in advance. If planning meals is difficult for you, try an online meal planner like Meal Mixer (www.mealmixer.com) or Meals Matter (www.mealsmatter.org). These resources can help to make customizing your menu plan, shopping list, and recipes a quick, simple, and easy task.

Principle #102

Don't skip breakfast.

You have probably heard people say that breakfast is the most important meal of the day, and that is true. Because we've spent the last 8 to 10 hours or so fasting during the night, we start the day low on fuel. Eating a healthy breakfast of lean proteins, fiber, and complex carbohydrates gives our metabolism a jump-start and fuels us for the day ahead. A simple, healthy breakfast, such as a hard-boiled egg, an orange, and whole grain cereal with low-fat milk, will energize you throughout the day and help prepare your body to receive and burn calories. Studies have shown those who enjoy a healthy breakfast are less likely to succumb to midday hunger that results in overeating.

Principle #103

Pass on the bread and chips when eating out—have soup or salad instead.

Bread, chips, and other snacks that are placed on the table for you to eat as you wait for your meal are tempting but contain little to no nutritional value. Often these snacks are packed with calories and fat. Instead of snacking on these empty calories, order a low-calorie soup or salad while you wait for your main entrée. A recent study showed that people who ate vegetable soup before their meal consumed 134 calories less at the meal. Likewise, the people who ate a salad consumed 12 percent fewer calories at the meal. So find a healthier alternative to the bread basket to curb your appetite.

Principle #104

Limit alcohol consumption and avoid "empty calories."

Robert C. Atkins, creator of the Atkins Diet, recommended refraining from alcohol consumption because "alcohol, when taken in, is the first fuel to burn." This means that while your body is burning alcohol, it is not burning fat. In addition, alcohol, at nearly 7 calories per gram, contains nearly twice as many calories per gram as carbohydrates and protein (4 calories per gram), and nearly as many calories as fat (9 calories per gram). These nutrient-deficient or "empty" calories quickly become fat if not burned off immediately. Decreasing the frequency and quantity of alcoholic beverages that you consume can greatly improve your health and assist in weight loss.

PRINCIPLE #105

Skip refined flour and sugar and avoid a crash.

Refined flour and sugar will give you a short burst of energy, but will inevitably culminate in a crash. Refined sugar is found in soda, cereal, sweets, honey, and high-fructose corn syrup. Refined flour, which is very low in fiber, is found in enriched breads and cereals, white rice, pasta, instant potatoes, and French fries To make healthier choices, opt for naturally occurring (unrefined) sugars that are found in fruits, vegetables, and milk. Or, eat whole foods, which are high in fiber, including whole wheat breads, pasta, and brown rice; oats; beans and peas; and vegetables. Avoid processed and refined foods and replace them natural and whole foods to give your body prolonged energy.

Principle #106

Eliminate junk food from your diet.

Junk food is food with little or no nutritional value. Often extremely processed, you'll know you are eating junk food when there is a long list of chemical-sounding ingredients on the nutrition label. Junk food often yields a temporary feeling of increased energy, but in reality it leaves the body weak and depleted. Often high in calories but low in nutritional value, junk food cause spikes in your blood sugar and a resulting withdrawal period. This withdrawal leads to decreased performance because of low blood-sugar levels and increases in sugar cravings. Cavities, obesity, heart disease, and type-2 diabetes have been linked to eating junk food.

Principle #107

Enjoy a colorful variety of fruits and vegetables.

An excellent way to ensure that you are getting a healthy selection of low-in-fat fruits and vegetables is to divide them into categories by color, as fruits and vegetables that share similar colors share similar nutrients. For instance, red fruits and vegetables, such as beets, red apples, tomatoes, and radishes, are colored by lycopene, which may help reduce the risk of several types of cancer. Orange/yellow fruits and vegetables are colored by carotenoids; beta-carotene, found in sweet potatoes and carrots, is converted to vitamin A, which promotes better eyesight. So enjoy an assortment of fruits and vegetables and reap the healthy benefits.

Principle #108

Know that a carbohydrate-restrictive diet will limit energy for exercise.

Although low-carb diets have become popular in recent years, complex carbohydrates are important for getting fit. Carbs are absorbed by the body and used as energy, thus, a lack of carbs can lead to physical and mental fatigue. Studies have also shown that without adequate carbs, your body will burn muscle protein to make energy. In other words, your body will begin breaking down the very muscle you are trying to build to use as fuel. Your meals should concentrate on complex carbs, such as fruit, vegetables, and whole grains, which are digested slowly by the body and help promote regular blood-sugar levels.

Principle #109

Give your body a break—avoid processed and prepackaged foods.

Your body is constantly working to break down food, process nutrients and vitamins, and create energy; however, processed and prepackaged food are very difficult for the body to break down and should thus be avoided. Processed and prepackaged foods often contain refined sugars, extra salt, and flavor enhancers, which can dull your taste buds to natural flavors. Processed food is also full of chemical additives, which enhance their color and keep them "fresh" longer. Finally, during processing much of the enzymes and nutrients of foods are stripped away, so your body won't benefit from the vitamins and minerals those foods would normally contain.

Principle #110

Schedule your meals
for the same time every day.

Your body has a natural daily cycle that is crucial to food digestion. Switching your meal schedule confuses your body, causing it to release digestive agents that create feelings of hunger. To prevent strong feelings of hunger, which could result in overeating, maintain a regular eating schedule. This will allow you to properly digest food and will help keep your blood-sugar levels more consistent throughout the day, keeping you from feeling starved come mealtime. Studies also show that people who eat on a consistent schedule tend to have lower caloric intake per meal compared to those who eat irregularly.

Principle #111

Eat your last meal by 6 p.m.

The body slows down at night, meaning that your metabolism won't be working as hard to burn calories. By eating your last meal of the day by 6 p.m., you not only eat when your metabolism is still high, but you give your body adequate time to digest the meal. After 6 p.m., avoid snacking in front of the TV while you are winding down from your day. If you are up late and find yourself ravenous, make your midnight snack a low-calorie bowl of whole grain cereal and low-fat milk, instead of ice cream or a slice of pizza.

Principle #112

Check the Nutritional Facts label to make smarter food choices.

A Nutritional Facts label appears on most foods, with the exception of meats and poultry. These labels offer information necessary for making smart food choices, including serving size; calorie content; and the content of fat, calcium, sodium, carbohydrates, fiber, and other nutrients. When you check these labels, you are better equipped to make healthy choices by limiting your intake of saturated fat, sodium, and cholesterol. For instance, we can now choose foods with lower fat, cholesterol, or sodium content, and which might be acceptable for a special diet. Read the nutritional label and make better food choices based on your food's nutritional value.

Principle #113

Eat high-quality foods and prepare them in healthy ways.

Eating high-quality foods and cooking them in healthy ways ensures that your body has the essential nutrients it needs to function at an optimal level. Start with foods with little or no chemical additives and avoid frying them or cooking them with oils and breading. Instead, prepare your food in a healthy manner: eat it fresh, baked, steamed, or grilled. Healthy, high-quality food prepared in these ways allows the natural flavors and nutrients to come out. You are what you eat, so don't drown your food in grease or strip it of its taste. Prepare your food in healthy ways to bring out the natural flavors and supply your body with the nutrients it needs.

Principle #114

Avoid eating large meals.

With desk jobs, computers, and automation, our lifestyles have become increasingly sedentary over the past several decades; unfortunately, our meals and their caloric values have increased. This disparity between what we need and what we eat has resulted in a nation of overeaters. To get fit and make significant advances toward your weight-loss and fitness goals, limit the size of your meals and the amount of calories you consume per meal. Studies have shown that individuals who eat large meals gain more weight than individuals who consume the same amount of calories in more meals.

PRINCIPLE #115

Eat smaller meals more frequently.

Experts recommend that those who want to lose weight may benefit from eating an increasing number of meals throughout the day. Rather than eating 3 bigger meals and 2 snacks, try eating 5 mini-meals. Eating smaller meals more frequently throughout the day forces your digestive system to stay active for longer periods, therefore, you will burn more calories. A quick and easy way to plan meals is to think in terms of halves. For instance, eat half of your lunch at noon and then enjoy the other half 3 hours later. Remember, when you increase the number of meals you eat per day, be sure to maintain the same number of calories.

PRINCIPLE #116

Be conscious of portion size when cooking at home.

Don't derail your hard work in the gym by eating huge portions when you cook at home. When you cook, set aside the amount of food that is equal to 1 serving, according to the Nutritional Facts label. Avoid eating in front of the TV or while you're busy with other activities, which can lead to overeating. Eat slowly, savoring each bite and its flavors so your brain receives the message when your stomach is full. If you must go back for seconds, choose from the low-calorie portions of the meal, choosing another helping of green vegetables and salad instead of meat and starchy foods. With some practice you'll be able to eyeball a healthy portion when you cook at home.

Principle #117

Take a daily multivitamin or mineral supplement.

Experts recommend that everyone take a daily multivitamin or mineral supplement that includes essential vitamins and minerals. A daily supplement can improve your physical and mental health as well as your overall bodily functioning. Vitamins and minerals are substances your body needs in small but steady amounts for normal growth, function, and health. It can be a challenge to get all the vitamins and minerals we need from food. Multivitamin and mineral supplements are an excellent and inexpensive "insurance policy" to vitamin and mineral deficiency. Check with your health care provider to see which supplements are best for you.

Principle #118

Include Omega-3 fatty acids in your diet.

Omega-3s are unsaturated fatty acids that are important to healthy cholesterol levels, proper blood flow, and healthy nervous system and heart functioning. Omega-3s are related to fitness, because they help your heart to perform during long cardiovascular exercise and to recuperate faster after vigorous strength training. The human body cannot synthesize Omega 3s; therefore, these fatty acids must be acquired as a dietary supplement or in the foods we eat, such as cold-water oil fish (salmon, mackerel, anchovies, and tuna), flax (flaxseeds and flaxseed oil), eggs, and walnuts.

Principle #119

Beware of frozen meals.

The frozen-food aisle in your grocery store is packed with frozen meals that claim to be healthy, convenient ways to lose weight. However, many of these meals, while low-calorie, are full of fat and sodium. When choosing healthy frozen dinners, check the serving size and nutritional values. Look for meals with less than 400 calories, less than 8 grams of fat, and less than 800 mg of sodium. Opt for the frozen meals that contain the most vegetables, offer brown rice or other whole grains, and use lean chicken or fish. Always choose carefully when buying frozen meals—not all are healthy options.

PRINCIPLE #120

Be conscious of portions while eating out.

Research shows that the more often a person eats out, the more body fat he or she has; this is because restaurants often serve portions that are large enough for 2, even 3 meals. To avoid overeating, share your meal with your dinner companion, order a half-portion, or order an appetizer as your main course. You will probably find that half the amount of food is more than satisfactory. Another great idea is to eat until you are full, and then take the rest of the meal home. You'll stop yourself from overeating, and have lunch for the following day! You might even ask for a portion of your meal to be boxed up right from the start, so you won't be tempted to eat more than you need.

Principle #121

Slow down to eat less.

A recent study of 30 normal-weight, college-age women revealed that when they ate quickly they consumed nearly 100 more calories than when they ate slowly. On average, the fast eaters in the study consumed 646 calories in about 9 minutes and the slow eaters ate about 579 calories in 29 minutes. It takes time for the stomach to relay signals to the brain, specifically that the stomach is full. Eating slowly allows the brain to catch up to the stomach. If you have eaten an amount of food that should be satisfying, but you are still hungry, wait 15 to 20 minutes before choosing to eat more. It is likely that, in that time, your brain will get the message that you are full.

Principle #122

Drinking green tea may improve your overall health.

Experts believe that green tea can vastly improve your health and decrease the risk of disease. Green tea is reported to contain the highest concentration of polyphenols, a powerful antioxidant. Antioxidants search for and neutralize free radicals, damaging compounds in the body that cause cell death, and alter DNA and cells. Green tea has been widely used in traditional Asian medicine for centuries and is said to prevent everything from headaches to cancer. An additional benefit for fitness enthusiasts is that green tea is a known natural appetite suppressant. So trade your morning coffee for a cup of iced or hot green tea and reap the health benefits.

Principle #123

Satisfy emotional needs through methods other than food.

The 5 typical emotions or states that cause overeating are loneliness, boredom, anger, stress, and fatigue. Those who are thin are able to catch themselves when eating out of emotion and stop before they overeat. If you are truly hungry, have a 100- to 200-calorie snack like a teaspoon of peanut butter on whole wheat toast. You should feel a boost in your energy right away. Find non-food related ways to satisfy emotional needs. Stay connected with friends and family who know you are trying to get fit. Exercise to relieve stress and curb emotional eating.

Principle #124

Fortify your body with calcium.

Calcium can increase the rate at which you lose weight. Three to four servings of low-fat dairy a day has been linked to reduced body fat. Though calcium supplements have also been shown to aid weight loss, the calcium from low-fat dairy produced higher levels of fat burning. If you cannot tolerate milk products, try other food sources of calcium, such as dark, leafy greens, salmon, almonds, or oatmeal. Calcium supplements should be combined with vitamin D, zinc, and magnesium, which helps increase the absorption rate. Aim for 1,000 to 1,300 mg of calcium daily to burn more fat.

Principle #125

Contact a medical professional if you have or have had an eating disorder.

Eating disorders are a serious matter. If you currently have or have had a history of eating disorders, please contact a medical professional before beginning any new diet and fitness plan. Certain foods and stress can trigger a response within you that can lead to binge eating, purging, and starvation. The stress of losing weight or making significant alterations to your diet may increase unhealthy compulsions. Consult with a doctor before starting any diet plan to help minimize the chance of relapse.

Staying Hydrated

All bodily functions use water in some form. Water comprises more than two-thirds of our bodies and is the base of all of our major organs and more than 85 percent of our brains. We use it to regulate body temperature, process and dispose of waste products, and facilitate chemical reactions at the cellular level. Water is second only to air in importance to the human body.

Proper hydration is the easiest and one of the most effective ways to bolster your body's immune system, improve physical performance, and prevent disease and illness. Dehydration on the other hand makes your body susceptible to fatigue, hunger, and, surprisingly enough, water retention.

Educate yourself about the benefits of hydration and learn how to maintain proper hydration so you can improve your performance and overall fitness. For instance, the human body can survive for weeks without food, but will die after only a few days without water. Even with this stark reminder of the importance of maintaining proper hydration, we often simply forget to drink an adequate amount of water.

Maintaining hydration is of significant importance when you are taking part in an exercise routine. This is because when you work out, you quickly lose water through perspiration. It is important to increase the amount of water you consume during your workouts to improve the overall function of your body and to help supply your muscles and vital organs with oxygen. Also, water can help support weight loss and help improve strength and endurance; the more water you drink, the more prepared your body is to effectively burn calories and to convert fat into energy.

While we all have different fitness goals and programs, drinking water is essential to our success. Not only will we look and feel healthier when we are well hydrated, but insufficient hydration can damage our bodies and negate the beneficial effects of working out. Examine the following principles to determine how much water you should consume and how you can maintain proper hydration.

Principle #126

Drink water; it is the most essential element for your body.

Water is the base of all major organs and constitutes more than two-thirds of the weight of the human body. Without water, a human being would die in just a few days. The human brain is 95 percent water, our blood is 82 percent water, and our lungs are 90 percent water. If our body's water supply drops just 2 percent, we'll see the signs of dehydration: headaches, a drop in short-term memory, lack of concentration, and constipation. Do you feel fatigued during the day? The most common cause of daytime fatigue is dehydration, and an estimated 75 percent of us suffer from it. No matter who you are, water is an essential element for your bodily functions.

Principle #127

Maximize your fitness performance through proper hydration.

No matter what your fitness goals are, they can be improved by staying properly hydrated. That's because just a 2 percent loss in water supply can lead to a 20 percent decrease in energy levels. Because it helps relieve conditions such as body aches, indigestion, and stress, proper hydration may contribute to long-term energy as well. In addition, every cell and organ in our bodies depends on water to function. For instance, water is the base of saliva, forms the fluids surrounding our joints, serves as a lubricant, regulates our body temperature through perspiration, and regulates metabolism. So, enjoy the benefits of water and maximize your fitness performance.

PRINCIPLE #128

Determine your ideal daily water intake.

Weight and metabolic rate determine how much water you should consume in a 24-hour period. Experts suggest that, in general, men should drink around 120 ounces of water per day, while women should have about 90 ounces per day. However, the amount of water required for each individual is determined by weight and metabolism. To calculate your ideal minimum water consumption, divide your weight (in pounds) in half. The resulting number is the amount of ounces of water you should consume. For instance, according to this calculation, a 180-pound person should drink about 90 ounces per day.

Principle #129

Stay hydrated in water-depleting circumstances.

Remember to take extra precautions and increase your water consumption when you are working out in temperatures above about 80 degrees or in high humidity. Very hot climates lead to risk of dehydration. If you are planning to work out in a dry climate where sweat evaporates quickly, drink an electrolyte-enriched drink. In such instances, increase both your overall hydration and the frequency at which you re-hydrate yourself. When engaged in activities or special situations that require a greater amount of hydration, it is recommended you carry a water bottle. The more accessible water is, the more likely you are to drink it.

Principle #130

Limit caffeinated drinks.

Caffeinated beverages, like coffee, tea, and soda are actually diuretics, which increase fluid loss. For this reason, you should limit the amount of caffeinated beverages you drink and adjust water consumption to compensate for fluid loss if you do drink these beverages. A simple way to ensure that you are drinking enough water is to drink a cup of water each time you refill your coffee mug. Try this simple tip: For every cup of coffee you have, drink 8 ounces of water This will help you offset the water loss and maintain proper hydration.

PRINCIPLE #131

Drink water before, during, and after each workout session.

When you work out you lose water rapidly through perspiration. In the hour prior to working out, you should drink between 8 to 16 ounces of water. While you workout, you should drink 4 to 8 ounces of water every 15 minutes. During vigorous cardiovascular training, or if you are exercising in hot temperatures, increase your water consumption even more. After working out, replenish your body by drinking between 8 to 16 ounces of water within 30 minutes of completing your exercise routine. Drinking the proper amounts of water post-workout will help reduce muscle soreness and will help your body recover.

PRINCIPLE #132

Drink fluids to supply your muscles and vital organs with oxygen.

Dehydration can cause a decrease in the amount of water in the blood. This reduction in blood volume inhibits the amount of oxygen in the bloodstream and may cause muscle fatigue, loss of coordination, and cognitive function. Also, blood pressure falls when a person becomes dehydrated. The body cannot adequately cool itself and there is a lack of blood and nutrients supplied to the body. Initially, you may become dizzy or have a foggy feeling come over you during or after working out. If this happens, take a seat and drink at least 12 ounces of water.

Principle #133

Avoid dehydration by drinking water before you feel thirsty.

---- ❋ ----

Dehydration weakens you, making your body more susceptible to fatigue, injury, and illness. However, symptoms come on gradually. It can take more than an hour for the effects of dehydration to be felt in your body. More obvious signs of dehydration, such as feeling thirsty and having dry mouth, usually occur after you have been dehydrated for a prolonged period. The initial signs can be more subtle and harder to detect. They often appear in the form of hunger pangs. If you have recently eaten and become hungry, drink a glass of water and wait 10 minutes. Chances are that you were actually thirsty, not hungry.

Principle #134

Drink more water to lose weight.

Weight loss experts suggest that water consumption may be the foundation of a successful weight-loss program. Therefore, by increasing the amount of water you consume, you may facilitate your weight loss. It's suggested that to lose weight, you drink an additional 12 ounces above the normal recommendations for your current weight, usually about six to eight 10-ounce glasses per day. Water directly benefits weight loss in quite a few significant ways: it maintains proper kidney function, which increases your liver's fat-burning ability; it is a natural appetite suppressant; it reduces water retention; and it helps the body function at optimal levels, making it easier to burn fat.

Principle #135

Avoid impaired physical and mental performance from dehydration.

Water is an essential part of every function of your body. When you are dehydrated during physical exertion, your body can no longer provide sufficient water to maintain both proper cardiovascular performance and body-heat regulation. It begins to ration the water it uses, slowing down and decreasing both your physical and cognitive abilities. Water also plays a key role in preventing disease. Recent studies have shown that those who drink at least 8 glasses of water a day have a decreased risk of colon, bladder, and even breast cancer.

Complementing Fitness with Nutrition

The foods we eat affect our bodies in significant ways. For instance, food can make us sluggish, energetic, raise our metabolisms, or cause rapid weight gain. Because foods vary in both their organic make-up and the manner and efficiency in which our bodies process them, it is important to create a diet of foods that will help us reach our personal goals of physical fitness. However, as a general rule, in order to boost your physical fitness and raise metabolism, it is better to choose foods that the body processes slowly.

Learn about the importance of diet to physical fitness. Choose a plan that works for you, and educate yourself about the nutritional values of everyday foods. You will see many more improvements far more quickly with a fitness-enhancing diet than if you fail to practice healthy eating.

Perhaps you are vegetarian or diabetic; perhaps you would like to gain weight or lose weight. Whatever your personal circumstances, create a diet that maintains basic nutritional requirements and promotes fitness advances. For instance, increase the amount of protein you eat for improved strength training. To improve cardiovascular fitness and muscle endurance, include more whole grains and complex carbohydrates in your diet.

When you eat will also affect your fitness goals. For instance, when strength training, it is beneficial to eat complex carbohydrates a half-hour to an hour before working out.

Examine how the foods you choose can help you reach your fitness goals. Learn how to implement a diet plan rich in healthy foods to achieve heightened results. The following principles will inform you about the effect specific foods have on your body. They will illustrate how you can choose healthier alternatives to your food cravings, and will also give you tips to bolster your body's metabolism in order to lose or gain weight while you enhance your physical fitness.

Principle #136

Create a diet containing proper nutrition to reach optimum fitness.

You will see few improvements to your body if you fail to practice healthy eating. A proper diet is essential to improving your overall health and to reaching a higher fitness level. If you want to make significant changes to your physical condition, first examine how your diet can help reach your goals. There are many types of diets, including vegetarian diets, high-protein diets, low-carbohydrate diets, low-sodium diets, macrobiotic diets, and so on. Choose a diet plan that works for you and that teaches you the proper foods to eat at the right portions for your specific circumstances.

Principle #137

Learn proper caloric intake for an appropriate diet.

Calories are a measurement of energy of which there are 2 types: the small calorie and the large calorie. The large calorie (or kcal) is the one we commonly use to measure food energy. One food calorie is defined as "the amount of digestively available food energy (heat) that will raise the temperature of 1 kilogram of water 1 degree celsius." The daily recommended calorie intake is 2,500 kcal/d for men and 2,000 kcal/d for women. Physically inactive people, children, and the elderly require less energy; while physically active, people require more energy.

PRINCIPLE #138

Burn 3,500 calories to lose 1 pound.

Your body creates calories through the digestion of food, and stores energy it does not use in the form of fat. These stored fat deposits feed your body when you are at rest or unable to eat. Some body fat is healthy, however, if the amount of calories you consume is greater than the amount of calories you use, over time your weight will be in an unhealthy range and you will need to lose pounds. To lose weight, you must create a calorie deficit where your body uses more calories than you consume. It takes approximately 3,500 excess calories to gain a pound; conversely, you must burn about 3,500 calories to lose a pound. Your metabolism and weight can increase or decrease this number.

Principle #139

Burn calories through everyday activities.

You can make small choices in your everyday life to significantly increase the amount of calories you burn in a day. For example, walking up a flight of stairs instead of taking an elevator, or parking at the far end of the parking lot and walking to a store will burn extra calories that would otherwise have been stored as fat. What about making little changes that most people don't even think about, like getting up to change the channel instead of using the remote? These minor changes to typical activities in your daily routine may seem small and unimportant; however, taken together, they culminate in burning significantly more calories per day.

Principle #140

Eat healthy foods that provide proper nutrition while avoiding excess calories.

For optimal health and fitness, it's important to eat foods rich in energy and essential nutrients and to avoid excess calories. Foods best to limit are alcohol, sugar, and saturated fats, as these are essentially packed with empty calories that lack nutritional food value. Excess calories are easily converted into fat, cause a decrease in metabolic function, and a loss of energy. The math of healthy eating is simple: to maintain your healthy goal weight, the calories you take in must be equal to the calories you put out; to gain weight, you must ingest more calories than you burn; and to lose weight, you must burn more calories than you ingest.

Principle #141

Eat complex carbohydrates to raise your metabolism.

Complex carbohydrates help you burn more calories, which results in accelerated weight loss. Complex carbohydrates can be found in foods like bread, cereal, rice, pasta, tortillas, crackers, pretzels, beans, and starchy vegetables (corn, potatoes, yams, peas, and plantain). Whole fruits, because of their fiber content, are also considered complex carbohydrates. Whole foods contain all of their nutrients and fiber, which naturally improve your body's digestive system and boost metabolism, whereas even "enriched" refined foods, contain only 5 nutrients (4 B vitamins and iron).

PRINCIPLE #142

Feel full longer and build lean muscle mass when you eat lean proteins.

Similar to fats, you'll feel full for a longer period of time by eating protein. Try to include 1 serving of a lean, protein-rich food such as skinless poultry, fish, egg whites, low-fat or fat-free milk products, beans, nuts, or tofu, with every meal. These types of food, when eaten along with your strength-training program, encourage the growth of lean muscle mass. The healthiest ways to prepare meats and poultry are baking, broiling, and roasting; for fish it's poaching, steaming, baking, or broiling. If you're in a hurry, try a high-protein drink or energy bar. Just make sure it is low in saturated fats and hydrogenated vegetable oils.

PRINCIPLE #143

Eat healthy snacks to bolster metabolism and stave off temptation.

Studies show that eating more frequently helps promote weight loss by increasing your body's metabolism. Snacking throughout the day, rather than eating 3 large meals, can be an effective way to eat more frequently. It can also be a recipe for disaster if the only snacks around you are high-calorie chips, cookies, and ice cream. There are lots of nutritious, low-calorie snacks, such as frozen fruit bars, yogurt, veggie soup, baked potato chips, and apple sauce, that if kept close at hand (in your desk, pantry, and car) can help stave off the temptation to eat empty-calorie snacks.

PRINCIPLE #144

Maintain steady blood-sugar level to enhance cardiovascular training.

Foods that will stabilize your body's absorption of nutrients, while providing level energy, help maintain you over long periods of a cardiovascular workout. These types of foods should provide steady energy throughout a training session. Select slow-burning carbohydrates, such as potatoes, oatmeal, and brown rice, so that you are better able to maintain blood sugar at a steady level. Avoid sugars and other fast-burning carbohydrates because they often lead to energy crashes in the middle of a session. An ideal meal consisting of complex carbohydrates should be eaten 1 to 2 hours before workout.

PRINCIPLE #145

Eat meals consisting of proteins for strength training.

Strength-training programs require energy and muscle-building nutrients if they are to be successful. Your meals should contain enough calories so that your body is able to perform the entire strength-training workout, but not so many that you will feel loaded down and lethargic. As a matter of fact, your body needs 1 gram of protein per pound of body weight to build and maintain muscle. Great sources of protein include red meat, poultry (chicken breast, turkey), fish (tuna, salmon, mackerel), eggs (including the yolk!), and dairy (milk, cottage cheese, yogurt). Meals packed with protein should be eaten 30 to 90 minutes before a session.

Principle #146

Replenish your body quickly after workout sessions.

Without proper post-workout nutrition, you may not see optimal results and might even undo some of the benefits of your workout. The proper post-workout meal can boost your metabolism and help your muscles strengthen and heal. These meals should be carbohydrate- and protein-rich with very little fat, as fat will slow down the digestion process. Post-training meals should take place immediatcly after completion of your workout session, because this is when your body is prepared to convey nutrients directly to the depleted muscles. The longer you wait to replenish nutrients, the less effective they are at reaching the targeted muscles.

Principle #147

Know both the risks and benefits of taking exercise supplements.

Usually in the form of pills, gels, and energy drinks, energy supplements and performance enhancers are over-the-counter products that use caffeine and other stimulants to boost your heart rate in order to maximize energy output during workout sessions. While you may benefit from improved endurance, concentration, and coordination in the short-term, the long-term benefits and problems have not been fully researched. Supplements may lead to dehydration and serious health complications. They may be dangerous to individuals whose heart is under strain. Do not take energy and performance enhancers without first consulting with your doctor.

PRINCIPLE #148

Carefully consider the use of creatine supplements.

Creatine is a chemical found naturally in the body that transfers energy to the muscles. It is often taken as a dietary supplement to improve muscle performance during high-intensity strength-training workouts. However, there is debate over the use of creatine supplements. Negative side effects may include muscle cramping, gas, bloating, and kidney stones. The effect of creatine on the heart muscle is as of yet unknown. Those considering using creatine should first consult their doctor.

Principle #149

Carefully consider the use of glutamine supplements.

Glutamine, found in raw parsley and spinach, is a conditionally essential amino acid. Vital to the body's production of proteins, it helps build and maintain muscle, aids in digestion, and assists the immune system. Highly concentrated in the muscles, glutamine can be severely depleted during intense strength training, leaving you susceptible to muscle depletion, illness, and other health problems. People with kidney problems, cirrhosis of the liver, Reye's Syndrome, pregnant women, and women who are breast-feeding should not take glutamine supplements.

PRINCIPLE #150

Consider taking protein supplements.

Protein is the most essential element for building strong muscles. Many people choose to take some of their protein in the form of supplements, usually powders and shakes that are designed to increase the amount of protein in your body without adding fat. There are different types of protein supplements to choose from, including whey protein (highly popular protein), whey isolate (powerful whey protein), micellar casein (slow-digesting protein), egg protein (good protein source), and soy protein (healthy protein choice). Protein powders and shakes have little risk of side effects. However, increased caloric consumption, especially in concentrate form, may lead to an increase in body fat.

Principle #151

Eat fiber to facilitate
weight loss and aid digestion.

Studies have shown that a diet rich in fiber will help decrease hunger sensation and allow the body to feel full longer. Fiber keeps the appropriate amount of water in your intestines. This helps your digestive system process your food more efficiently and keeps your bowel movements regular. Studies have also shown that increased fiber in your diet may decrease your risk of colon cancer, ease the effects of diabetes, and prevent stroke and heart disease. Fiber is readily available in fruits, nuts, vegetables, beans, and whole grains.

Principle #152

Avoid diets that deny your body proper nutritional value.

Diets that do not include proper nutritional value deny your body of the fuel and building materials it needs to maintain healthy functioning. Improper nutrition can deplete your body of energy, break down muscles, and undo the beneficial effects of your fitness routine. Consider how different foods affect your body in order to choose a diet that helps you reach your fitness goals. Identify which foods provide you with essential nutrients and how these nutrients improve your overall bodily functioning.

Principle #153

Avoid crash diets, which slow your basal metabolic rate.

Your body's basal metabolic rate (BMR) is the amount of energy you use when your body is at rest. It is the energy needed just for the functioning of your vital organs, muscles, and skin, and it is measured when your digestive system is inactive, about 12 hours after eating. Your BMR typically represents about 70 percent of all calories consumed. However, when you maintain a regular fitness routine and eat properly, you have a higher BMR. In other words, you essentially burn more calories even while your body is at rest. Conversely, if you undergo crash diets and forgo exercise, your BMR slows down, which will result in decreased weight loss.

Principle #154

Don't skip meals if you want to lose weight.

One of the biggest misconceptions is that skipping a meal will result in greater weight loss. However, the exact opposite is true. Skipping meals or eating too little, can slow or stop your weight loss. There are a few reasons for this: the biggest one being that skipping meals causes your metabolism to slow down, which means you burn fewer calories, thus sabotaging your goals. Another important reason is that when you skip meals it can lead to being extra hungry later. When you get too hungry you lose your will power to eat healthy portions and foods and are far more likely to binge and overeat, again resulting in defeating your weight-loss plans.

Principle #155

Eat low-density, high water-content foods to fill you up without weight gain.

Studies show that low-density foods with high water content allow you to eat until you're full and still lose weight. These foods include such healthy, high-fiber choices as non-starchy vegetables, high water-content fruits, fat-free milk, chicken and veggie broth, fruit, fiber, fish, and lean proteins. Because these foods have low calorie content and high water content, you can eat more of them. As a result you get full, but consume fewer calories. Fill up on high-fiber fruits, vegetables, and whole grain foods. These foods, including grapefruit, broccoli, apples, have been shown to help boost the efficiency of your digestive track and steady insulin levels.

PRINCIPLE #156

Fuel workouts with monounsaturated and polyunsaturated fats.

Fat is critical to a healthy diet and is an excellent source of fuel for your workouts. However, there are good fats (monounsaturated and polyunsaturated fats) and bad fats (saturated fats). Your body can burn good fats as fuel. Good fats lower total cholesterol and LDL (bad) cholesterol while increasing HDL (good) cholesterol. Common sources of good fats include salmon; corn, soy, safflower, sunflower, canola, and olive oils; olives; avocados; and nuts. Limit saturated fats, which your body can't burn as fuel. Saturated fats are found in animal products, such as meat, dairy, eggs, and seafood, as well as coconut, palm, and palm kernel oils.

Principle #157

Pass on "diet foods" in favor of a real meal.

Many supposed "diet foods" contain appetite-stimulating artificial sweeteners that can actually make you hungry. For instance, the sweetener Aspartame, more commonly known as NutraSweet, which is most frequently found in diet sodas, is a neurostimulant that has been linked to stimulating the appetite. In addition, while diet foods may suppress hunger in the short-term, they often fail to provide long-lasting energy, leading to an increase in food cravings and diet fatigue. Whenever possible, eat a real meal, keeping diet foods for occasional snacks or for when you're on the go and are unable to enjoy a proper meal.

Principle #158

Avoid diets where you eat large amounts of protein to lose weight.

Traditionally, diets designed to increase muscle mass have promoted a high-protein diet. Generally, these diets recommend that you consume much more protein than you actually need for daily functioning. If your goal is to gain muscle, you can generally expect to consume 1.2 to 2 grams of protein per each pound you weigh. Above this amount, you are just consuming excess calories that will lead to weight gain over time if they are not burned off during exercise. Also, high amounts of protein can flush your body of water. If additional fluids are not taken in to compensate for excess protein intake, you may experience a decrease in your performance.

Principle #159

Time your meals to improve workout performance and results.

When building muscle mass, both what and when you eat are important. Experts recommend that you eat a meal rich in complex carbohydrates 30 to 60 minutes before working out. This will ensure proper energy levels throughout your workout. It's also recommended to eat a protein-rich meal within 30 minutes of completing your workout. This will help repair and build new muscle. Properly scheduling meals to coincide with your workout session will help your body reach a higher level of fitness.

OPTIMIZING FITNESS
FOR MAXIMUM RESULTS

When beginning a workout routine, it is important to formulate a fitness strategy by first establishing your goals and then determining the means by which you will accomplish them. Before beginning your program, lay out a plan or strategy that will be your path to improved physical fitness.

Start with a visualization exercise. When you visualize your new body, what does it look like? Are you interested in gaining muscle mass or are you looking to become more toned and have increased endurance? Whatever your desired outcome, studies have shown that your body will become physically stronger and healthier when you partake in a fitness program.

Once you've decided the type of training you will engage in, it's time to decide when, where, and with whom you will be training. There are 4 primary options to choose from when creating a fitness program: (1) a gym, (2) a personal trainer,

(3) at home, and (4) group training. Each of these choices has both benefits and restrictions. Examine your personal fitness goals and personal preferences before selecting the option that is right for you.

Whatever strategy you choose for your personal fitness plan, it's important to know your limitations. Avoiding injury is dependent on pacing yourself, learning proper technique, and having the proper form when doing any type of physical fitness training. You will also want to stop working out if you feel any pain. Though there will be days when you feel muscle soreness, you should never feel severe pain.

The most important factor is whether the system will not only fit into your current lifestyle, but that it is something you will look forward to doing day in and out. Staying motivated can be half the battle of your fitness goals. You might choose to use music, a pedometer, or heart monitor to inspire you; or you might commit to a workout buddy or personal trainer.

The following principles address the strategies of choosing, maintaining, and enjoying your physical fitness routine.

Principle #160

Commit to a workout partner.

There are lots of reasons to commit to a workout partner. First off, you are committed to someone besides yourself. Many people find that this added commitment gets them to the gym even when they don't want to go. A workout partner will help encourage and motivate you to follow through on your fitness goals, and working in tandem with someone else can help you pace and track your results. Most of all, working out with a partner is fun. It makes time fly by and takes the focus off just getting through your workouts. There are many online resources to find workout partners, including www.exercisefriends.com and www.readytosweat.com.

Principle #161

Choose a gym.

Gyms come in many forms, from local gyms, such as independent or university-affiliated gyms, to national chains such as Bally's, 24 Hour Fitness, and the YMCA. When you are searching for the right gym, take into account its proximity to your home and place of business, as well as the cost and hours and amenities it provides. Most gyms will allow prospective members to workout a few times as a trial for free or at day-pass rates. Go to the gym during the hours you would normally work out and see if you feel comfortable there before deciding to join.

Principle #162

Reach your goals
with a personal trainer.

Working out with a personal trainer is an excellent way to get fit. A trainer will teach you proper technique and use of machines, will help to motivate you through difficult times, and will also help you maximize your workout sessions. A trainer can help you reach your goals faster, track your progress, and manage your fitness routine. It is not only important to find a trainer who works well with you and with whom you get along, but also to find a trainer who is properly certified. A typical trainer will meet with you for about an hour, 1 to 3 times a week.

PRINCIPLE #163

Consider working out at home.

When you start your new fitness routine, you may find it too costly or uncomfortable to work out at a gym. If this is so, consider working out at home. There are many activities that you can do in your home and in your neighborhood. Outdoor activities such as running, hiking, and bicycling are an excellent forms of cardiovascular training, and home gym machines, weight sets, and rubber bands are very effective when strength training at home. You might even use ordinary household items like 1-pound bags of pasta and 5-pound bags of beans for strength training. However, when working out at home you must be vigilant and avoid the many temptations and distractions that you'll find there.

Principle #164

Learn something new in a group exercise class.

Group exercise is a fun and exciting way to work out. Classes are usually held in a large workout room, similar to a dance studio, and can include cardio work, strength, and flexibility training, or a combination of all three. Classes are usually 1-hour long, set to music, and include a warm-up and cool-down. With the variety of classes that are available today, you are sure to find one that suits your needs and is appropriate for your level of fitness. Ask for a schedule of classes at your local gym or pick an activity that interests you and search the Internet for classes in your area. Whatever your flavor, you're sure to find a group exercise class that suits you.

PRINCIPLE #165

Use music as an excellent motivator.

Studies in sports psychology have consistently proven that music is a source of motivation and inspiration for sport and exercise participants. Many people find that by including music in their fitness routine, their workout sessions are more enjoyable and even more productive. Download your music to an MP3 player or other device and let the rhythm of your favorite tunes push you during your cardiovascular and strength-training sessions. Listening to music can motivate you to relieve stress and push yourself further during your workouts.

Principle #166

Stretch at your desk.

Sad but true, many of us are deskbound daily, and worse, we use it as an excuse not to exercise. Stretching exercises are a natural for those of us who sit all day. Ease stress and keep your muscles from clenching by doing stretching exercises in your chair. Here are 2 simple exercises you can try. To stretch your back, sit tall in your chair, stretch both arms over your head, reach as high as you can for 10 seconds. Extend first the left hand higher then the right hand higher. Repeat. For your neck, roll your head gently to the right, so that your ear almost touches your shoulder. Hold for 10 seconds. Repeat on the other side.

Principle #167

Prepare for setbacks and obstacles.

Though much of the time it is, exercise is not always easy and fun. There will be times when you can't make or don't want to make a workout, times when you have to have that chocolate bar, and times when life just gets in the way. It can be easy to use the blame you feel to justify quitting your program entirely. Instead of falling into the failure trap, give yourself credit for every step you take toward health and fitness, no matter how small it may seem to you. Prepare yourself mentally for setbacks and obstacles to your health and fitness program by knowing there are no good reasons to quit. Just try again tomorrow.

Principle #168

Use a pedometer or heart monitor to track your workout.

Many people find that by using a pedometer or heart monitor, they can more accurately track the results and efficiency of their workouts. Using a pedometer (or step counter) allows you to record the number of steps you take, and they can be encouraging motivators as you see the steps add up each day. Step counters are being put into MP3 players and mobile phones. Usually consisting of 2 elements, a chest strap and a wrist receiver, heart monitors track and measure your heart rate, which is very helpful when you are training toward certain cardiovascular goals. For better results, track your workout with one of these devices.

Principle #169

Learn proper mechanics of gym and fitness equipment.

It is important to understand the purpose and proper function of fitness equipment in order to avoid improper use and possible injury. Don't be afraid to ask gym employees or other patrons to explain to you how a machine or piece of fitness equipment works. When using equipment for the first time, read the instructions on the side of the machine and go slowly in order to avoid injury. Pay attention to your form as you work out and you will make more substantial long-term gains in your physical fitness.

Principle #170

Know your limitations.

Avoid injury by knowing your limitations and by taking all the necessary precautions before you start your workout. Remember, don't overexert yourself, especially when you first begin an exercise program. Learn proper technique and form before performing exercises with large amounts of weight, and pay close attention to the instructor in group exercise classes. Pace yourself and work with a partner or spotter when training with heavy free weights. Avoid pushing yourself too hard at the start of a fitness routine. Maintaining a fitness routine is a lifelong endeavor, so don't rush your body. Know your limitations and slowly expand them.

Principle #171

Enjoy the social benefits of a team sport or group exercise class.

Joining a fitness group or team sport is an excellent way to exercise and the social reinforcements will help you stay motivated. When you become a member of a team you are not only responsible to yourself, but your teammates are also counting on you. You will be less likely to skip a workout session if it means that your team will be placed at a disadvantage or forced to forfeit. Team sports are an excellent way to exercise and have a good time while you do so. Your business may have a company softball or basketball team, and many gyms have leagues you can sign up for as an individual or with a group of friends.

Principle #172

Evaluate your current medical condition before beginning any fitness routine.

Know the shape you are in before you begin any fitness routine. It is important to make sure your body is healthy enough for your fitness routine. Take into consideration your current level of activity, previous medical conditions, and other limiting factors. If you have ever been told by a medical professional that you have a heart condition; if you have recently experienced chest pains, loss of balance, or loss of consciousness; if you become dizzy as a result of physical activity; or if you know of any other reason why you should not do physical activity, contact a medical professional before beginning your exercise program.

Principle #173

Stop making excuses and find solutions instead.

Excuses are the enemy of getting fit. They give you a reason to stop doing what you know is good for you. In order to better prepare yourself for the excuses that will inevitably come up, write them down, then write down how you plan to overcome them. For instance, if a common excuse is "I don't have time to exercise," devise a plan to walk for 20 minutes during your lunch break. If another excuse is "I'm too tired," find a workout buddy who can motivate you, even after a long day. Find solutions and your excuses for skipping workouts will fall by the wayside.

Principle #174

Build your fitness routine
to reach individual goals.

When creating your workout plan, consider what you are trying to achieve. Your goals will determine the type of activity, intensity, frequency, and duration of your workouts. If your goal is to lose weight, you will probably want to focus on cardiovascular activities, balancing them with strength and flexibility training. Similarly, if you want to gain weight and build muscle mass, you will need to focus on weight training, while still incorporating cardio and flexibility training. Take into account your age, current health, fitness level, personal interests, and work schedule when creating your fitness routine.

Principle #175

Limit strength-training sessions to 1 hour or less.

When a muscle is worked for a long duration, the focus of the exercise will automatically shift from increasing power to increasing endurance. A muscle will react in order to adapt to the stress it is submitted too. When you strength train for long periods of time, the dominant stress shifts from the resistance of the weight to the amount of repetitions performed. The muscle will subsequently adapt in a way that helps increase muscle endurance at the expense of power. So, if your goal is to build muscle mass, limit your strength-training sessions to 1 hour or less.

Principle #176

Allow 2 days rest between strength-training sessions.

Resting is an essential part of strength training. Allow 2 days rest between strength-training sessions so that your muscles have time to rest and heal after your workouts. You will fail to make great improvements in your overall performance and may make yourself more susceptible to injury if you do not allow your muscles time to recuperate. As a matter of fact, studies have shown that decreasing rest between workout sessions may not only fail to increase your performance but it may actually decrease your muscles' strength.

Principle #177

Stop working out if you feel pain, sickness, or dizziness.

It is very important to remember that if you feel pain, ill, or very dizzy, stop working out immediately. It is possible to injure yourself during strength, cardio, and flexibility training sessions. If you are working out and feel pain, sickness, or dizziness, don't try and push through it. When you strength train, you should never feel sharp or prolonged pain during or after your workouts. Sickness or dizziness can be due to dehydration. If you feel uncomfortable, stop, sit down, and drink water. Always listen to your body.

Principle #178

Schedule your workout routine to match your lifestyle.

Many people find that by working out in the morning, they experience a boost in energy throughout the day. Many others find that exercising in the early evening helps prepare them for sleep. You should select the routine that best suits your lifestyle. Do not try to conform to a specific schedule, rather, allow your natural tendencies and lifestyle to determine your schedule. You may choose to work out during your lunch hour some days, after work other days, and early in the morning on the weekends. All are great options. When you select a routine that fits nicely into your lifestyle, you are more likely to maintain it and allow it to become part of your life.

Principle #179

Consider an online personal trainer.

A low-cost alternative to hiring a personal trainer is to use one who you find on the Internet to help track your workouts and provide expertise. These trainers will help you select appropriate exercise routines for your lifestyle and fitness goals, and they will help you track your results via email or text messaging. Due to the proliferation of Internet trainers, it is important to find one who is a certified personal trainer. For beginners and fitness novices, it is recommended that you schedule at least a few in-person sessions with your personal trainer in order to learn about proper form, use of equipment, and healthy eating.

Maintaining a Healthy Lifestyle: Helpful Tips

Each and every one of us can reap many benefits by incorporating health and fitness into our lives. The rewards of a healthy lifestyle don't stop at finally fitting into our favorite outfit again. They are sometimes even more noticeable when we can do what we haven't been able to in so long. For instance, when we can play a game of softball with our kids without getting winded, or when we can climb a flight of stairs with ease.

Of course, a healthy diet and exercise program can also be the key to better sleep; better moods; decreased depression, anxiety, and stress; and a reduced risk of heart disease.

When you switch your perspective and begin to see fitness not as a destination, but rather as a path you will travel for a lifetime, the do-or-die attitude you may have toward fitness disappears and in its place is real change. This chapter provides motivating and helpful tips that you can use to enhance your existing healthy lifestyle and improve your overall fitness.

For instance, if you are having difficulty setting goals for yourself, try working toward a fitness event. Knowing that you are working toward a goal can often be the deciding factor in working out today.

In addition, this section contains information that is specific to certain groups of people (such as pregnant women or people with asthma). Physical fitness can and should be an important part of your life despite physical limitations or other special circumstances. Often those who benefit the most from physical fitness routines are those who may have some form of limitation. Even if these tips do not apply to you, review them because they may apply to a friend or loved one. Once you become fit, you will feel an overwhelming desire to help others reach fitness goals.

The following principles will help you optimize your health and fitness plan for a lifetime.

Principle #180

Consult your doctor to be sure you can maintain your fitness plan.

Before beginning any fitness routine, consult your doctor. He or she will have advice on how you can exercise in a way that is both safe and beneficial for your body over time. Your doctor will also help you avoid activities that may be harmful to your particular situation. He or she will tell you if you suffer from high blood pressure or have any other conditions that might require you to limit your workout. If you've been sedentary for a prolonged period, your doctor may advise you to take it easy until you've adjusted to your new regimen. Follow your doctor's advice and get the most benefit out of your fitness program.

Principle #181

Take care of your feet;
invest in quality exercise shoes.

Select supportive exercise shoes with adequate cushioning, as poorly fitting footwear can result in discomfort, blisters, and serious injury. Replace shoes if you experience aches or pains in your feet, knees, legs, hips, or lower back. In general, running shoes should be replaced every 4 to 6 months; all-purpose athletic shoes should be replaced once a year. When purchasing exercise shoes, visit a specialty footwear store where they will measure the length, width, and arch of your foot to fit your shoes properly. While at the store, you should walk around, run in place, and jump to check the fit. The more comfortable your feet are, the more you will enjoy your workouts.

Principle #182

Wear proper clothing.

When working out, wear clothes that are not too constricting and that allow for your body's full range of motion. Clothes should be made from breathable materials that stretch and move when you do. It is important to enjoy your workout clothes, as they can give you the extra bit of incentive you might need to work out on days when you're not feeling like it. Fitness clothes can be expensive. If possible, don't worry too much about the price; you will get more use out of your workout clothes than any other outfit in your wardrobe.

Principle #183

Understand that setbacks are not failures.

Do-or-die attitudes to fitness are a surefire way to set you up for failure. This type of perfectionist mentality leads to frustration if you miss workouts, hit plateaus, and fall off your diet plan. There will be times when you feel you are not reaching one of your goals; allow for these setbacks, as it is the only way to grow. Remember, these aren't really failures, they are opportunities for growth! Learn from them. Avoid creating unrealistic goals as these are destined to be unreachable. Plan for some setbacks, enjoy your successes, and concentrate on long-term growth as you make real, lifelong changes in your health and fitness habits.

Principle #184

Be honest with yourself.

Don't lie to yourself. If you cheat on your diet or overindulge, admit to it. If you skip a workout or do the bare minimum one day, acknowledge it. The only way you will ever replace negative habits with better ones is by first accepting that they do actually exist. Lying to yourself and making excuses will only hurt you and keep you from reaching your goals. Give yourself a break— we all have times that we don't stick to our plans. Just take a breath, accept the facts, resolve yourself, and get back on track.

PRINCIPLE #185

Get inspired to make positive changes in other areas of your life.

Many people find that success in transforming themselves physically has a collateral effect on other aspects of their lives. Studies show that the increased confidence and self-esteem brought on by achieving fitness goals, enhanced mood from taking part in exercise, and a more balanced eating plan, can enhance your abilities in other areas of your life. You may choose to engage in new social engagements that you would have found intimidating in the past. As a result of your newfound confidence you may choose to seek out a new job, ask for a raise, or even ask someone out on a date. The possibilities are endless when you feel inspired by success.

Principle #186

Keep a food journal.

Keeping track of what you eat and drink and monitoring your food decisions, emotions, and hunger levels is crucial to your weight-loss success. A food journal can be a highly effective daily reminder that helps you stay focused on your personal goals and keeps you motivated toward your weight-loss target. You will be able to keep track of your food and beverage intake, make sure you are within your daily calorie allotment, and ensure that you are getting enough fluids. You should also log your physical fitness activities, supplements, energy levels, and daily weight. This ongoing routine will make it easier to lose weight.

Principle #187

Relieve the physical and emotional strain of pregnancy with exercise.

Working out may offer both physical and emotional benefits to pregnant women. Exercise may help relieve excessive weight gain, swelling of hands and feet, leg cramps, varicose veins, insomnia, fatigue, and constipation. Many gyms offer yoga and aquatic exercise for moms-to-be. These low-impact activities decrease the risk of injury to you and your baby. After giving birth, enjoy mommy-and-me classes at your local gym. These can be a great and healthy way to bond with baby. Remember, if you are pregnant, it is extremely important to contact your doctor before beginning any fitness routine.

Principle #188

Don't view hunger
as good or bad.

Hunger is just your body's natural signal to fuel itself. People tend to read into their hunger more than they need to. Thin people look at hunger as a simple signal from their bodies that they need food for energy. Most people who carry extra weight view hunger as a condition to be avoided. Therefore, overweight people consistently overeat or eat when they don't have any natural signals. Thin people recognize their hunger and understand where these sensations are coming from. If you find yourself eating for no reason, try skipping a snack. You may realize that you didn't even need it.

Principle #189

Improve your asthma with regular exercise.

Research shows that most asthmatics would benefit from regular physical activity; many people with asthma, however, fear that exercise is not an option for them. Studies have shown that many asthmatics can build up a tolerance for physical exertion over time. According to ACE, the American Council of Exercise, the following exercises are listed in order from most to least likely to induce an asthma attack: outdoor running, treadmill running, cycling, walking, and swimming. If you have asthma, talk with your doctor before beginning any fitness routine, and be sure to have a fast-acting inhaler with you whenever you work out.

Principle #190

Get your body in motion and it will want to remain in motion.

Your body not only needs exercise to function well, it actually craves it. With every workout session, your desire to be physically active will increase. With time, your stamina will improve and your energy will increase as a result of a routine exercise program. As your conditioning improves, your heart and breathing rates will return to normal resting levels much more quickly after strenuous activity. As exercising gets easier, your body's need to keep moving will spread to other areas of your life. The confidence you feel and the abundance of energy you have will encourage you to pursue new adventures. Your overall lifestyle will improve as a result of exercise.

Principle #191

Make a New Year's resolution to start your fitness routine before the holidays.

Every January 1, millions of Americans pledge to lose weight, only to give up soon after. Traditionally, people vow to lose weight as a sign of contrition for the weight they've gained during the holiday season. This year, take a different tack. Start your New Year's resolution in early November to make real lasting change. When the holidays arrive, you will be practiced at avoiding temptation, eating healthily, and exercising regularly. Successfully navigating the holidays will give you the confidence you need to maintain your program in the new year.

Principle #192

Keep a bag packed.

If you always have a bag of workout gear ready to go, you'll never succumb to an excuse like, "I don't have my running shoes so I can't go to the gym today." Better still, you'll be in a position to accept invitations for exercise, such as an impromptu hike or Pilates class. Keep a bag packed with workout clothes, socks, running shoes, a light jacket, a swimsuit, a water bottle, and sunscreen in your car or at your office. When you drive by an inviting hiking trail or a friend suggests a bike ride after work, you will have everything you need right at your fingertips!

PRINCIPLE #193

Know that walking is an effective way to incorporate daily exercise.

Don't think you have to sprint for 30 minutes each day to get an effective workout; in fact, as we've said, overexerting yourself is dangerous. The truth is, both low- and high-intensity exercises have equal potential for burning calories and helping you lose weight. A daily walk is a great way to incorporate exercise into your routine. When you don't have time for a serious gym session, take a brisk walk around your neighborhood. For instance, a 180-pound person will burn about 100 calories per mile—a great way to burn extra calories and make sure to get fitness in daily.

Principle #194

Make it known that fitness is your priority.

While sharing your desire to get fit with your friends and family creates a network of support, it is also important to make it clear to your loved ones that fitness is a very real priority in your life. Everyone has a person in their life who, albeit innocently, tries to get them off track when it comes to diet and exercise. This might be an aunt who pushes a second piece of pie at you during the holidays, or a coworker who suggests you skip the gym in favor of after-work cocktails. Be strong and firm when you stick to your nutrition and fitness plan. You won't offend anyone by making it clear that your priority is getting fit and being healthy.

Principle #195

Luxuriate in the decreased stress of your everyday life.

Exercise provides an opportunity to relieve emotional tension. In addition, working out releases endorphins, which promotes an overall feeling of happiness and well-being. The confidence you build with exercise also reduces stress. And, finally, exercise provides an opportunity to be social, which is great for reducing tension. So be sure to enjoy the decreased levels of stress you experience because of regular exercise! Luxuriate in a better night's sleep and more calm energy throughout your day. Once you start experiencing the relaxation exercise brings, you will crave even more physical activity.

PRINCIPLE #196

Get plenty of sleep.

Sleep is critical to optimal body and mental functioning. As a matter of fact, it is so critical that you will spend about one-third of your life doing it. If you do not get adequate rest, your body attempts to compensate for low energy levels by craving sugar and carbohydrates that will give it a quick burst of energy. Sleep allows your body to heal properly; it helps decrease stress levels and improves your mental outlook. Sleep helps facilitate muscle growth and increased muscular strength, and it is an essential aspect of proper bodily function. Without proper sleep you cannot reach your optimum fitness levels, so for your health and fitness, enjoy 7 or 8 hours a night.

Principle #197

Select a large fitness event and work toward it.

Working toward a fitness event is a great way to train. Check your local gym or sports supply store for a list of events in your area. Start with a 5k run or 20k bicycle ride and work your way to bigger events like a half-marathon or mini-triathlon. Train slowly by yourself or with a group. Many charities raise donations with fitness events, for instance the Avon Walk for Breast Cancer and the Dr. Seuss Walk for Literacy. Participating in these events will not only give you a goal to work toward that will improve your fitness; it will also raise funds for a worthy cause.

Principle #198

Replace your mid-morning coffee with a 10-minute walk for increased energy.

Caffeine will give you a quick jolt of energy that will quickly fade and leave you tired again and craving more caffeine. Replace your mid-morning coffee with a vigorous, 10-minute walk around the building. You will feel invigorated and rejuvenated when you return to your desk. Your legs and arms will enjoy the increase in blood circulation and your mind will appreciate the change of scenery. A brisk walk around the building will refresh you, leaving you more alert and focused for the work at hand.

Principle #199

Surround yourself with individuals who share your fitness goals.

Avoid slipping back into a sedentary lifestyle by surrounding yourself with people who share fitness goals similar to yours. Use your new active lifestyle to engage in social activities with people who share similar mentalities on fitness. Those around you have a big influence on your activities, and friends who share your interests will help motivate you when you're feeling sluggish or down. In addition, they'll be grateful when you return the favor.

Principle #200

Enjoy yourself!

Although it will require hard work, health and fitness should be fun! Choose healthy foods, exercises, and activities that appeal to you. Find friends who share your interests. Create an environment where you look forward to working out. Plan meals full of healthy foods you enjoy. Reward yourself at each milestone. If you begin to dread going to the gym or out for a walk, change your routine. And if you slip up or fall off your diet and exercise routine, don't worry. Just get back on the program the next day. There are endless possibilities for fun with health and fitness, so enjoy exploring them all!

Additional
Information and Ideas

The information in this section is created to help you build an effective fitness plan.

First, you can review several charts that will help you determine your current physical condition and goals for a fitness program. You will be able to assess your current heart rate, blood pressure, and body composition, and, in turn, use these same figures to see your progress over the course of your fitness efforts.

Second, answer a series of important questions about your fitness history, current condition, obstacles, diet choices, and goals. Evaluating your answers to these questions can help you create realistic fitness goals, target attitudes, and assess your progress along the way.

Evaluating Your Current Condition

While the clearest results of maintaining a regular fitness routine are visible, often the internal improvements are more significant. Excess body fat and a sedentary lifestyle can significantly damage your body and put you at risk for diseases, such as type-2 diabetes. Examine the following charts in order to determine your current and goal conditions.

Heart Rate

Heart rate is a leading indicator of your baseline fitness level and can be used as a guide to maximize the results of cardiovascular exercise. The heart is a specialized muscle that is designed to pump the blood needed to maintain all of your bodily functions. Blood brings oxygen and nutrients to every part of the body. A heart's performance is essential to maintaining every aspect of a body down to the cellular level. Your heart rate is the number of times your heart beats in a minute. This number is a clear indicator of the efficiency of your heart. A strong heart pumps more effectively with each contraction and therefore doesn't need to beat as fast to supply the body with blood. A high heart rate indicates that the heart is not as efficient at circulating blood and therefore needs to pump faster to keep up with your body's needs. As your heart becomes better at pumping blood through regular exercise, you will find that your heart rate will decrease. Use these numbers to determine your current fitness level.

Resting Heart Rate Fitness by Age and Gender

Men by Age Group:

Heart Fitness Level	18 –25	26 –35	36 –45	46 - 55	56 -65	65+
Excellent	50-60	50-61	51-62	51-63	52-61	51-61
Good	61-68	62-69	63-69	64-70	62-70	62-68
Average	69-76	70-77	70-78	71-79	71-78	69-75
Fair	77-80	78-80	79-81	80-83	79-80	76-78
Poor	81+	81+	82+	84+	81+	79+

Women by Age Group:

Heart Fitness Level	18 –25	26 –35	36 –45	46 - 55	56 -65	65+
Excellent	55-64	55-63	55-63	55-64	55-63	55-63
Good	65-72	64-71	64-72	65-72	64-72	64-71
Average	73-80	72-78	73-80	73-79	73-79	72-79
Fair	81-83	79-81	81-83	80-82	80-82	80-81
Poor	84+	82+	84+	83+	83+	82+

Blood Pressure

It is important to determine your blood pressure before starting a physical fitness program in order to establish baseline health. Those suffering from high blood pressure should contact a medical professional before beginning any physical fitness routine. Blood pressure is the force of blood against the arteries created by the heart as it pumps blood through the circulatory system. Like all muscles, the heart cycles between being active and inactive, therefore blood pressure varies accordingly. Systolic blood pressure refers to the pressure when the heart is pumping. Diastolic pressure refers to the pressure when the heart is at rest. Blood pressure is recorded with these 2 numbers and usually referred to as the systolic number over the diastolic (e.g., 130/90). The following table lists risk categories and corresponding blood pressure ratings.

Blood Pressure Table

SYSTOLIC	DIASTOLIC	STAGE AND HEALTH RISK
210	120	High Blood Pressure/Hypertension Stage 4/Very Severe Risk
180	110	High Blood Pressure/Hypertension Stage 3/Severe
160	100	High Blood Pressure/Hypertension Stage 2/Moderate Risk
140	90	High Blood Pressure/Hypertension Stage 1/Mild Risk
140	90	Borderline High
130	90	High Normal
120	85	Normal – Optimum
110	75	Low Normal
90	60	Borderline Low
60	40	Low Blood Pressure – Hypotension
50	33	Very Low Blood Pressure – Extreme Danger

Body Composition and Body Mass Index (BMI)

The body functions best when it consists of a proper proportion of muscle, fat, organs, and bone. Your body composition is determined by the ratio of these elements against the body's mass. While bone and organ mass and weight remain relatively constant, fat and lean muscle varies from individual to individual. The percent of body weight that is made up of fat and lean muscle is an important indicator of body composition and overall fitness. Without proper amounts of both muscle and fat the body will fail to work at its optimum. Your Body Mass Index (BMI) is also an excellent source for determining the condition of your heart and its risk for cardiovascular disease. Examine the chart on the following page to determine your body composition and risk for cardiovascular disease.

Body Mass Index (BMI)

Height	Minimal Risk Normal Body Weight (BMI 19-24)	Moderate Risk Overweight (BMI 25-29.9)	High Risk Obese (BMI 30 and up)
4'10"	91-115	119-142	143 or more
4'11"	94-119	124-147	148 or more
5'0	97-123	128-152	153 or more
5'1"	100-127	132-157	158 or more
5'2'	104-131	136-163	164 or more
5'3"	107-135	141-168	169 or more
5'4"	110-140	145-173	174 or more
5'5"	114-144	150-179	180 or more
5'6"	118-148	155-185	186 or more
5'7"	121-153	159-190	191 or more
5'8"	125-158	164-196	197 or more
5'9"	128-162	169-202	203 or more
5'10"	132-167	174-208	209 or more
5'11"	136-172	179-214	215 or more
6'0"	140-177	184-220	221 or more
6'1"	144-182	189-226	227 or more
6'2"	148-186	194-232	233 or more
6'3"	152-192	200-239	240 or more
6'4"	156-197	205-245	246 or more

Questions to Ask Yourself

Before you start a workout routine, ask yourself the following important questions in order to determine your current fitness level and your fitness goals. Review the questions and see how they pertain to you. You may want to write down your answers in a journal so that you can reference them later, or simply reevaluate your fitness goals as you go along.

Questions about your fitness history and current fitness level:

1. How old are you?
2. What is your height?
3. What is your weight?
4. When were you in the best shape of your adult life?
5. Have you ever participated in a workout program?
6. How long did you maintain the program?
7. What did the program include?
8. Why did you quit the program?
9. What led to you or inspired you to get into shape now?

10. What obstacles have kept you from meeting your previous fitness goals?
11. What steps are you going to take to ensure these obstacles do not inhibit you this time?
12. How many hours a week do you engage in physical exercise?
13. Rate your current fitness level on a scale of 1-10 (1=Worst 10=Best).
14. What is your resting heart rate?
15. What is your active heart rate?
16. What is your blood pressure?
17. What is your cholesterol?
18. What is your body fat percentage or BMI?
19. How many push-ups can you do (without pausing) before having to quit because of exhaustion?
20. How many pull-ups can you do (without pausing) before having to quit because of exhaustion?
21. How many sit-ups can you do in 1 minute?
22. How many squats can you do (without pausing) before having to stop because of exhaustion?

23. Can you touch your toes?

24. Do you smoke?

25. How many alcoholic beverages do you consume a week?

26. Have you ever been told by a medical professional that you have a heart condition?

27. Do you feel pain in your chest during physical activity?

28. Have you experienced chest pain in the last month when not engaged in strenuous physical activity?

29. Have you ever lost balance or consciousness because you became dizzy while undergoing physical activity?

30. Do you suffer from joint or bone ailments or injuries that may become exacerbated due to physical activity?

31. Are you taking prescription drugs for high blood pressure or another heart condition?

32. Do you know of any other reason why you should not do physical activity?

Questions about your new fitness routine:

1. What do you want to accomplish with your workout program?
2. What are the reasons you want to get fit?
3. What type of physical results do you want to achieve with your workout?
4. How long will you maintain this program (short-term)?
5. What is the start date?
6. What is the end date (short-term)?
7. What are your short-term goals?
8. What are your long-term goals?
9. What are the top 3 things you hope to get from your workout program?

Questions about fitness preferences:

1. What types of physical activities do you enjoy and why?
2. What types of physical activities do you dislike and why?
3. Do you prefer to exercise alone, with a partner, or in a

group and why?

4. What time of day do you have the most energy? What time of day would you be most likely to work out?

5. What kinds of obstacles (physical and mental) would prevent you from exercising?

6. Describe your cardiovascular-training program.
   a. How many training sessions do you plan per week?
   b. How long will each session last?
   c. What types of activities do you plan on doing?

7. Describe your strength-training program.
   a. How many training sessions do you plan per week?
   b. How long will each session last?
   c. What types of activities do you plan on doing?

8. Describe your flexibility-training program.
   a. How many training sessions do you plan per week?
   b. How long will each session last?
   c. What types of activities do you plan on doing?

9. What fitness classes or groups might you join?

10. What type of clothes will these activities require?

11. How many times a week do you want to work out?

12. What days of the week do you have available for exercise?
13. How will you schedule fitness into your weekly routine?
14. How will you warm-up and cool-down for each workout?
15. What is your contingency plan if your original workout plan becomes too strenuous or time-consuming?
16. If you are planning to exercise outside, do you have a contingency plan for bad weather?
17. How will you measure your progress?
18. How long do you think it will take to reach your goal?

Questions about current diet and eating habits:

1. How often do you eat fried foods?
2. How many times a week to you eat fast food?
3. How often do you eat fruit/vegetables?
4. How many glasses of water do you drink a day?
5. How many caffeinated beverages do you have a day?
6. Do you take a daily multivitamin?
7. How many meals a day do you eat?

8. Do you regularly eat breakfast?

9. Do you often skip meals?

10. Do you often eat large amounts of food after dinner, close to bedtime?

11. Do you eat while doing other activities (e.g., watching TV, driving a car)?

12. Do you eat more when under stress? Less?

13. Do you often indulge in sweets or fatty snacks?

14. Describe your nutritional program:

    a. What are your nutritional program goals?

    b. How many glasses of water will you drink daily?

    c. How many meals will you have each day?

    d. Will you take a multivitamin or supplement?

    e. How many calories will you consume daily?

Conclusion

Every year, millions of Americans spend billions of dollars buying get-fit-quick gimmick books and diet pills. These supposed miracle cures rarely make a difference and we are left frustrated and depressed. We think that it must be our fault. We read the testimonials and saw the before-and-after results on the infomercial, but we weren't able to do what they did. These fabricated tales of drastic weight loss capture our attention while distorting our perceptions of what real fitness should be.

By reading *Simple Principles® to Get Fit*, you have made the first important step toward educating yourself about personal fitness and dispelling the quick-fix myths. You have begun to change not only your body, but also your mind. You can now begin to create realistic and achievable fitness goals. Switch the focus away from the unhealthy, impossible images you see in the media and replace them with a personalized vision of a healthier and happier you. With hard work, dedication, and the principles presented in this book, you will make real, long-lasting changes. Working within your current lifestyle, you have learned how to target specific fitness goals and how you can more easily reach them through training and nutrition.

Reference this book often in order to keep these concepts fresh in your mind. Try not to view the principles in this book as rules that must be followed, but rather guidelines. The information in this book should teach you to think in a new way about fitness and help you make your own decisions about how you are going to live a healthier lifestyle.

Unfortunately, there is no magic pill that will let us shed 20 pounds overnight, but with dedication, hard work, and by following *Simple Principles® to Get Fit*, you can make real, lasting changes, and create a happier, fitter you.

TELL US YOUR STORY

Simple Principles® to Get Fit has changed the lives of countless people, helping them look, feel, eat, and work out better than they ever imagined. Now we want to hear your story about how this book has helped you get fit.

Tell us ...

- Why did you purchase this book?
- Which areas of your fitness or nutrition did you want to work on?
- How did this book help you improve in those areas?
- How did this book change your life?
- Which principles did you like the most?
- What did you like most about this book?
- Would you recommend this book to others?

Email us your response at info@wspublishinggroup.com or write to us at:

WS Publishing Group
7290 Navajo Road, Suite 207
San Diego, CA 92119

Please include your name and an email address and/or phone number where you can be reached.

Please let us know if WS Publishing may or may not use your story and/or name in future book titles, and if you would be interested in participating in radio or TV interviews.

Great Titles in the
SIMPLE PRINCIPLES™ SERIES

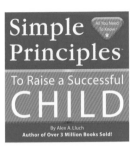

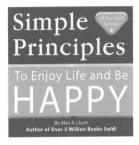

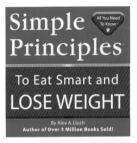

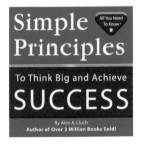

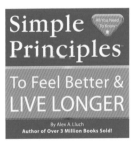

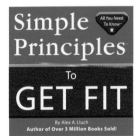

More Great Titles in the
SIMPLE PRINCIPLES™ SERIES

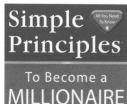

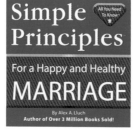

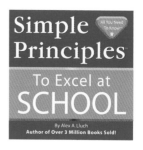

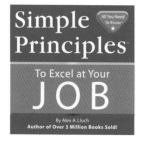

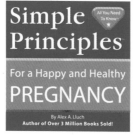

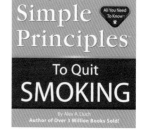

LOG ON TO **WSPublishingGroup.com** TO CHECK FOR
RELEASE DATES ON THESE AND FUTURE TITLES.

Other Best-Selling Books
by Alex A. Lluch

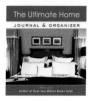

HOME & FINANCE
- The Very Best Home Improvement Guide & Document Organizer
- The Very Best Home Buying Guide & Document Organizer
- The Very Best Home Selling Guide & Document Organizer
- The Very Best Budget & Finance Guide with Document Organizer
- The Ultimate Home Journal & Organizer
- The Ultimate Home Buying Guide & Organizer

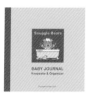

BABY JOURNALS & PARENTING
- The Complete Baby Journal Organizer & Keepsake
- Keepsake of Love Baby Journal
- Snuggle Bears Baby Journal Keepsake & Organizer
- Humble Bumbles Baby Journal
- Simple Principles to Raise a Successful Child

CHILDREN'S BOOKS
- I Like to Learn: Alphabet, Numbers, Colors & Opposites
- Alexander, It's Time for Bed!
- Do I Look Good in Color?
- Zoo Clues Animal Alphabet
- Animal Alphabet: Slide & Seek the ABC's
- Counting Chameleon
- Big Bugs, Small Bugs

LOG ON TO **WSPublishingGroup.com** TO CHECK FOR RELEASE DATES ON THESE AND FUTURE TITLES.

More Best-Selling Books
by Alex A. Lluch

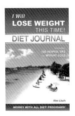

COOKING, FITNESS & DIET

- The Very Best Cooking Guide & Recipe Organizer
- Easy Cooking Guide & Recipe Organizer
- Get Fit Now! Workout Journal
- Lose Weight Now! Diet Journal & Organizer
- I Will Lose Weight This Time! Diet Journal
- The Ultimate Pocket Diet Journal

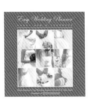

WEDDING PLANNING

- The Ultimate Wedding Planning Kit
- The Complete Wedding Planner & Organizer
- Easy Wedding Planner, Organizer & Keepsake
- Easy Wedding Planning Plus
- Easy Wedding Planning
- The Ultimate Wedding Workbook & Organizer
- The Ultimate Wedding Planner & Organizer
- Making Your Wedding Beautiful, Memorable & Unique
- Planning the Most Memorable Wedding on Any Budget
- My Wedding Journal, Organizer & Keepsake
- The Ultimate Wedding Planning Guide
- The Ultimate Guide to Wedding Music
- Wedding Party Responsibility Cards

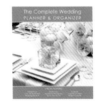

LOG ON TO **WSPublishingGroup.com** TO CHECK FOR RELEASE DATES ON THESE AND FUTURE TITLES.

About the Author and Creator of the
SIMPLE PRINCIPLES™ SERIES

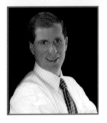

Alex A. Lluch is a seasoned entrepreneur with outstanding life achievements. He grew up very poor and lost his father at age 15. But through hard work and dedication, he has become one of the most successful authors and businessmen of our time. He is now using his life experience to write the Simple Principles™ series to help people improve their lives.

The following are a few of Alex's achievements:

- Author of over 3 million books sold in a wide range of categories: health, fitness, diet, home, finance, weddings, children, and babies
- President of WS Publishing Group, a successful publishing company
- President of WeddingSolutions.com, one of the world's most popular wedding planning websites
- President of UltimateGiftRegistry.com, an extensive website that allows users to register for gifts for all occasions
- President of a highly successful toy and candy company
- Has worked extensively in China, Hong Kong, Spain, Israel and Mexico
- Designed complex communication systems for Fortune 500 companies
- Black belt in Karate and Judo, winning many national tournaments
- Owns real estate in California, Colorado, Georgia and Montana
- B.S. in Electronics Engineering and an M.S. in Computer Science

Alex Lluch lives in San Diego, California with his wife of 16 years and their three wonderful children.